Laboratory Evaluation of Hemostasis and Thrombosis

Laboratory Evaluation of Hemostasis and Thrombosis

THIRD EDITION

MARJORIE S. SIRRIDGE, M.D.
Professor of Medicine
Director of Docent Hemostasis Laboratory
University of Missouri-Kansas City School of Medicine
Hematology Consultant
Providence–St. Margaret Health Center
Bethany Medical Center
Children's Mercy Hospital

REANER SHANNON, Ph.D.
Assistant Professor
University of Missouri-Kansas City School of Medicine

LEA & FEBIGER   •   1983   •   Philadelphia

Lea & Febiger
600 South Washington Square
Philadelphia, PA 19106
U.S.A.

Library of Congress Cataloging in Publication Data

Sirridge, Marjorie S.
  Laboratory evaluation of hemostasis and thrombosis.

  Rev. ed. of: Laboratory evaluation of hemostasis.
2nd ed. 1974.
  Bibliography: p.
  Includes index.
  1. Blood—Coagulation, Disorders of—Diagnosis.
2. Blood—Analysis and chemistry—Laboratory manuals.
3. Hemostasis. 4. Thrombosis. I. Shannon, Reaner.
II. Title. [DNLM: 1. Hemostasis. 2. Thrombosis.
WO 500 S6224L]
RC647.C55S57 1983   616.1'570756   82-21692
ISBN 0-8121-0878-7

PRINTED IN THE UNITED STATES OF AMERICA

Print Number 5 4 3 2 1

Preface

Since the second edition of this book was published in 1974, I have continued to see many patients with hemostatic problems and have become increasingly interested in patients with thrombotic problems. It is for this reason that the title of the book has been changed to include our experience with the laboratory investigation of the latter. I have continued to teach medical students and residents and medical technologists, and have worked with my coauthor, Reaner Shannon, to establish the Docent Hemostasis Laboratory at the University of Missouri-Kansas City School of Medicine.

My primary laboratory interest continues to be in those studies that can be performed accurately in the clinical laboratory and that are useful in the diagnosis of disease states and the care of patients. We have performed many new procedures and have done comparative studies in several areas to determine which procedures are the most accurate, convenient to perform, and economical. In this book, we have included primarily those tests with which we have personal experience and which we consider useful. It is so easy to initiate tests because they are fashionable and because kits are available that make the procedures seem less difficult. The ordering physician and the laboratory technologist must understand what a test is measuring, the principles of the method used, the accuracy of the method, and the relationship of the test to others that are being performed. The separation of the laboratory from the clinical arena has discouraged this joint responsibility.

New research in the areas of hemostasis and thrombosis has broadened and changed our understanding of hemostatic processes. In Chapter I, we have included much of this new information and have integrated it with older facts that are still accurate. I am sure the future will bring additional changes. Chapter II is greatly increased in length because of the explosion of clinical information about bleeding and clotting disorders. The remaining chapters, which relate to the techniques of testing, include remarks concerning the principles involved, the specific methods to be used, and discussions of how to use and interpret results. Many tests are based on clotting end points, but the availability of synthetic substrates and radioimmunoassay procedures has expanded and significantly changed the methodology of the hemostasis laboratory. We have made a major effort to standardize procedures and reagents, as well as the style of describing methods. The major equipment in our laboratory has not changed significantly since 1974.

I wish to thank Betty Steinman and the Audio-Visual Department of the University of Missouri-Kansas City School of Medicine for their invaluable help in the development of new illustrations for this edition. Also, for frustrating hours spent in typing this manuscript, I wish to thank my secretary, Gladys Burns. It has been a tremendous help to be able to share the responsibility of this edition with Reaner Shannon with whom I have now worked in the laboratory evaluation of hemostasis and thrombosis for 12 years. Much of the research work in the area of hypercoagulability which we have done in the Docent Hemostasis Laboratory has been supported by the Lettie V. McIlvain Trust.

MARJORIE S. SIRRIDGE, M.D.
Kansas City, Missouri

Nothing is more frustrating to a medical technologist than attempting to follow a test procedure and finding that all the details and directions are not provided or that the procedure is difficult to comprehend. This has been my experience on several occasions when trying to develop or implement new procedures from those described in the medical literature. Therefore, in helping to write this book, I have placed particular emphasis on procedural details. Every attempt has been made to be as clear, precise, and thorough as possible in describing all procedures in order to make it easier for those who wish to use them. I hope this objective has been accomplished.

I express my gratitude and appreciation to Dr. Marjorie Sirridge for the opportunity to share the authorship of this book and for the knowledge and experience I have gained in the years I have worked with her. I consider myself fortunate, for it is a rare opportunity to be associated with such an investigator and physician.

REANER G. SHANNON, M.T. (ASCP), Ph.D.
Kansas City, Missouri

Contents

CHAPTER *1*

Mechanisms of Hemostasis and Thrombosis

Blood is normally fluid; in the body it circulates throughout the vascular system under pressure. The prevention of spontaneous bleeding and the control of traumatic hemorrhage are referred to as hemostasis. Until recently, most research efforts related to hemostatic mechanisms were directed toward determining and studying those abnormalities that result in bleeding problems due to disturbances of hemostasis. It has become apparent, however, that far more important is the study of processes and changes that result in the formation of intravascular thrombi in intact, non-traumatized arteries, veins, and capillaries. This is referred to as thrombosis. Hemostasis is known to be dependent primarily on the following:

1. Normal resistance and contractility of blood vessels and an adequate supportive framework for them.
2. Normal platelet activity, which includes adequate numbers and function.
3. An adequate coagulation system.
4. Stability of the clot.

Vessels, platelets, and the coagulation system are all important in thrombus formation, which is the major mechanism for hemorrhage control. After vessel injury, the exact sequence of events is not always the same, and the following factors have been shown to be of variable importance.

1. Location of the injured vessels and the chance of continuing trauma (i.e. oral cavity, joints).
2. Size of vessels, flow patterns, and blood pressure within them; also the potential for contraction of the vessel wall.
3. Intrinsic abnormalities of the vessels.
4. Abnormalities or damage to surrounding tissues.
5. External pressure on vessels due to edema or hemorrhage into surrounding tissues.
6. Application of external pressure or surgical intervention.

For example, in large arterial vessels in which the blood pressure is high, usually the flow of blood cannot be slowed sufficiently to allow an occluding thrombus to form without the application of a tourniquet, the use of external pressure at the bleeding site, or some type of surgical intervention. Occasionally, enough tissue damage surrounds the vessel, with accumulation of blood in this tissue, to produce local tamponade of an artery with eventual cessation of bleeding. With repeated trauma, however, bleeding is easily reactivated. With the use of local pressure, hemostasis is more easily accomplished in large veins that have been traumatized than in large arteries; but usually some type of surgical intervention is also required. Local tamponade by accumulated blood in tissues is more effective in producing venous occlusion. In small venules and capillaries, hemostasis may be accomplished by the simple adhesion of endothelial surfaces and the local adhesion and aggregation of platelets with the deposition of stabilizing fibrin strands. In small arteries and arterioles, however, spontaneous control of bleeding requires a complex interaction among the components of the vessel wall, the platelets, and both the intrinsic and extrinsic pathways of coagulation for the formation of occluding thrombi (Figure 1-1).

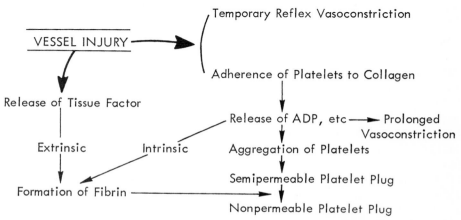

Figure 1-1.   Interrelationships in hemostasis in small arteries and arterioles.

Many of the factors involved in hemostasis are also important in the process of thrombosis. In large arterial vessels, there may be gradual narrowing of the lumens by the adherence of platelets and fibrin and the formation of atherosclerotic plaques, which can eventually result in the complete occlusion of these vessels by local thrombus formation. In the intact venous system, particularly in the lower extremities, the spontaneous formation of large venous thrombi is an important clinical problem usually related to altered flow patterns, resulting in stasis. Thrombi form in intact small arteries, veins, and capillaries due to local changes in vessels and to systemic stimuli, which may result in disseminated microvascular clotting.

The process of thrombus formation, which occurs during both hemostasis and thrombosis, usually proceeds in the following way:

1.   A change in the endothelium of the vessel.
2.   Adherence of platelets to collagen, basement membrane, and subendothelial microfibrils. (Fibronectin is an adhesive glycoprotein in connective tissue, which is required for normal platelet interaction with collagen.)
3.   Initiation of the platelet release reaction by collagen and other stimulating substances present at the site (within 3 seconds).

4. Further aggregation of platelets by ADP, thromboxane A_2, and other substances released from platelets with the formation of a reversible platelet plug.
5. Generation of thrombin, probably initially by the extrinsic pathway.
6. Further aggregation of platelets by thrombin, formation of fibrin by thrombin, and stimulation of clotting via the intrinsic pathway.
7. Formation of a stable fibrin-platelet plug (within 1 to 4 minutes).
8. Continued formation of fibrin by both extrinsic and intrinsic pathways.
9. Entrapment of RBCs and more platelets in fibrin strands with thrombus formation.
10. Eventual lysis or organization and recanalization of the thrombus.

As we have come to better understand the relationship of the hemostatic mechanism to thrombotic diseases, it has become important to examine how this process affects the blood vessel walls. During the thrombotic process, collagenase and elastase enzymes become available and alter the surrounding connecting tissue. Activated platelets release a factor that is mitogenic for smooth muscle in the walls of arteries and arterioles, and this may initiate the formation of atherosclerotic plaques. Chemotaxis of leukocytes occurs. When platelets go through the release reaction, vasoconstriction caused by the release of thromboxane A_2 (TxA_2) is initiated. This effect of thromboxane A_2 may be opposed by the release of prostacyclin (prostaglandin I_2, PGI_2) from endothelial cells, since PGI_2 is not only a potent inhibitor of platelet aggregation but also causes vasodilatation. With thrombus formation, plasminogen activator is released from the vessel wall and converts plasminogen in the thrombus to plasmin. If enough plasmin is formed, the clot will be lyzed; if not, it must be organized and recanalized. Most thrombi in the microcirculation are lyzed rapidly because of their small size; but in larger vessels, organization and recanalization are more likely to occur.

BLOOD VESSELS

When blood vessels are normal, blood cells are retained within them except when actual injury occurs; however, defects in structure, permeability, contractility, and resistance may interfere with adequate hemostasis and result in hemorrhagic problems. The recognition of such defects rests primarily on careful clinical observation rather than on laboratory studies. Clinical evaluation is made not only on observation of a bleeding area, but also on inspection of the surrounding tissues and the remainder of the patient's body for evidence of generalized disease that might affect vascular function.

Problems of thrombosis related to blood vessel structure are recognized primarily by invasive techniques such as venography and arteriography which allow visualization of the size, contour, and degree of abnormalities in the deep veins of the lower extremities, the pulmonary circulation, the aorta, the coronary, cerebral and renal vessels, and others. Noninvasive techniques such as impedance phlethysmography, Doppler studies, and radionuclide scanning have also been useful in the study of arterial and venous thromboembolic processes. With the advent of successful reconstructive surgery for some vascular abnormalities and the widespread use of anticoagulant and fibrinolytic drugs, it has become important to determine the presence and extent of such abnormalities to plan appropriate therapy.

PLATELETS

Normal hemostasis requires that platelets be present in adequate numbers and that they be capable of fulfilling several important functions. Abnormalities in number and function can result in both hemorrhagic and thrombotic problems. Platelets normally arise from the cytoplasm of megakaryocytes in the bone marrow and are delivered into the bloodstream. The number of available platelets is dependent on the productive capacity of the megakaryocytes in the marrow and their survival in the circulation, which is normally 8 to 12 days. The marrow reserve is not excessive and can be rapidly depleted

Platelets are structurally complex, and they undergo changes in shape when they come in contact with various stimuli. Such changes render them adhesive to exposed collagen at sites of vascular injury, a process that requires the presence of a plasma protein called Willebrand factor. This factor is part of the factor VIII molecule. Normal stimulated platelets then aggregate and release several substances (among them, adenosine 5'diphosphate; ADP) which are active in inducing further aggregation. These rapid early events are reversible, but with the continuing release of ADP and other substances, and the associated formation of fibrin, more aggregation takes place and the platelet aggregates become stabilized. During these processes, phospholipid compounds (referred to as platelet factor 3) are made available on the surface of platelets. These substances become integral components of several steps in the intrinsic pathway of coagulation. Platelets also release factor V which is important in the formation of thrombin.

The release reaction is energy-requiring and is due to the formation of the endoperoxides PGG_2 and PGH_2 from arachidonic acid, which is normally present in platelet membranes. From these endoperoxides, thromboxane A_2 (Tx_2) is formed, and its release with other substances from platelets mediates continued platelet aggregation and induces the contraction of the smooth muscle of the walls surrounding arterioles. Thus, by the adherence and aggregation of platelets at sites of vascular injury and the induction of local vasconstriction, there is a slowing of blood flow which allows the initiation of clot formation. Platelets also contribute to clot retraction through the attachment of their pseudopods to fibrin strands and a reaction between adenosine triphosphate (ATP) and thrombosthenin, the contractile protein contained in their cytoplasm.

COAGULATION SYSTEM

The coagulation system is by far the most complex part of the hemostatic mechanism and involves the interaction of 10 or more different factors from plasma an tissue, as well as the regulation of these reactions by natural inhibitors. Our present concepts of the workings of the system are the result of some simple observations and the sophisticated research studies of many investigators. Some basic facts that are important in understanding coagulation include:

1.   In a glass tube, blood clots in about 10 minutes.
2.   In a plastic or siliconized tube, blood may take as long as 30 minutes to clot.

3. If powdered glass or other activating substances are added to plastic or siliconized tubes, blood will clot in about 2 minutes.
4. Blood to which tissue extract has been added clots in a few seconds.
5. The clotting time of recalcified plasma is much shorter than that of whole blood and shows a variability that is at least partially dependent on the speed and length of centrifugation. Platelet numbers in plasma are also known to be affected by the manner of centrifugation.
6. The recalcification time of plasma can be reduced by adding a platelet substitute, an activator substance, or tissue extract.

From these and similar observations, the following conclusions can be drawn:
1. Normal blood contains all factors needed to form a clot.
2. Some factor or factors in blood must be activated by a contact, such as with a glass tube, and this appears to be a time-consuming process. Activation is less likely to occur when blood is exposed to plastic or siliconized surfaces.
3. The process of contact activation could not require calcium, since at least partial activation occurs in blood or plasma to which a calcium-binding anticoagulant has been added.
4. Tissue factor contains a substance or substances that bypass the contact-activation process.
5. Since platelets influence the speed of the clotting process to some extent, they must also be involved in the intrinsic coagulation system.

International Nomenclature of Coagulation Factors

An international nomenclature has been established for the coagulation factors. This should be mastered before trying to understand the probable manner in which these factors interact. Most factors are regularly referred to by number, with the exception of fibrinogen (I), prothrombin (II), thromboplastin (III), and calcium (IV), and several other more recently described factors (prekallikrein, high molecular weight kininogen, Passavoy). Table 1-1 designates the factors by number and/or name and includes some of the known facts that are important in studying and understanding their functions.

The coagulation factors may be conveniently divided into three groups: the fibrinogen family, the prothrombin family, and the contact factors (Table 1-2). The fibrinogen family consists of fibrinogen itself and the three cofactor proteins VIII, V, and XIII. All are of large molecular size (MW > 250,000) and, with the exception of factor VIII, are known to be synthesized in the liver. The prothrombin family is made up of the four vitamin K-dependent clotting factors, II, VII, IX, and X. All are made in the liver, are small molecules (MW 55,000 to 70,000), and can be converted into serine protease forms. Factors XII, XI, and prekallikrein are somewhat larger than the prothrombin family proteins (MW 80,000 to 200,000), and these serine protease zymogens become activated on contact. High molecular weight kininogen (HMWK) has a molecular weight of 110,000 and acts as a cofactor for the contact-activation reactions.

Intrinsic and Extrinsic Pathways

The generation of thrombin (factor II_a), which converts fibrinogen to fibrin, represents the central event in the coagulation of blood. This occurs as a result of a

TABLE 1-1.   International Nomenclature of Coagulation Factors

Factor Number	Names	Known Facts
I	Fibrinogen	MW 340,000 Synthesized in the liver T½—80–90 hours Heat labile and storage stable Concentration—2500–3500 μg/ml
II	Prothrombin	MW 70,000 (Protease) Synthesized in the liver T½—60–70 hours Heat stable and storage stable Vitamin K-dependent Concentration—100–150 μg/ml
III	Tissue Thromboplastin Tissue factor	High molecular weight lipoprotein Obtained from saline extraction of most body tissues Normally absent from plasma
IV	Calcium	
V	Proaccelerin Labile factor Accelerator globulin	MW 270,000 Synthesized in the liver T½—15–25 hours Heat labile and storage labile Concentration—5-15 μg/ml

VI	Accelerin—this factor is
	  no longer considered
	  in the scheme of hemostasis	

VII	Proconvertin Stable factor Serum prothrombin conversion accelerator (SPCA) Autoprothrombin I	MW 60,000 (Protease) Synthesized in the liver T½—5 hours Heat labile and storage stable Vitamin K-dependent Concentration—0.5 μg/ml

VIII	VIII:C
	  Procoagulant Activity
	    VIIIC:Ag—Immunologic
	VIII:R
	  Factor VIII Rel.Protein
	  VIIIR:Ag—Immunologic
	              Willebrand
	                 factor
	VIIIR:RCF
	          Ristocetin
	             cofactor
	Antihemophilic factor (AHF)
	Antihemophilic factor A
	Thromboplastinogen
	Platelet cofactor I
		MW VIII:C 285,000
		     VIII:R 85,000↔3,400,000
		Synthesis
		  VIII:C unknown
		  VIII:R endothelial cells
		T½—8–16 hours
		Heat stable and storage labile
		Concentration—15 μg/ml

IX	Plasma thromboplastin component (PTC) Christmas factor Antihemophilic factor B Autoprothrombin II	MW 55,000 (Protease) Synthesized in the liver T½—12–24 hours Heat labile and storage stable Vitamin K-dependent Concentration—3 μg/ml

Factor Number	Names	Known Facts
X	Stuart-Prower factor	MW 55,000 (Protease) Synthesized in the liver T½—40–45 hours Heat labile and somewhat stable on storage Vitamin K-dependent Concentration—10–15 μg/ml

XI	Plasma thromboplastin
	  antecedent (PTC)
	Antihemophilic factor C
		MW 160,000 (Protease)
		T½—64 hours
		Somewhat heat labile and increased on
		  storage
		Concentration—5 μg/ml

XII	Hageman factor (HF)	MW 80,000 (Protease) T½—40–60 hours Destroyed by heat to 60° C and storage stable Concentration—29–40 μg/ml
XIII	Fibrin stabilizing factor	MW 320,000 (Transpeptidase) Synthesized in the liver T½—120 hours Heat labile and storage stable Concentration—20 μg/ml
—	Fletcher factor Prekallikrein	MW 85,000 (Protease) Concentration—50 μg/ml
HMWK	High Molecular Weight Kininogen Fitzgerald factor Flaujeac factor	MW 110,000 Concentration—70—90 μg/ml
—	Passavoy factor	
AT III	Antithrombin III	MW 65,000 Synthesized in the liver T½—48 hours
—	Plasminogen	MW 90,000 Synthesized in the liver T½—2.2 ± 0.29 hours

TABLE 1-2.   Coagulation Factor Families

Fibrinogen Family	*Prothrombin Family*
Fibrinogen (I)	Factor II
Factor VIII	Factor VII
Factor V	Factor IX
Factor XIII	Factor X

(Large molecules,
  absent in serum)
	(Small molecules,
	  vitamin k-dependent)

Contact Factors
Factor XII
Factor XI
Prekallikrein
High Molecular Weight Kininogen

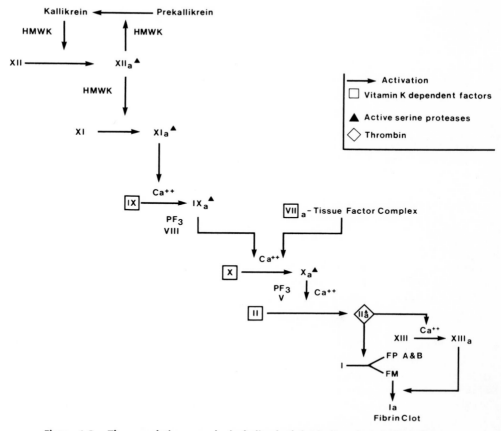

Figure 1-2. The coagulation cascade, including both intrinsic and extrinsic pathways.

cascade of sequential reactions involving coagulation factor enzymes (factors XII, XI, prekallikrein, IX, VII, X, II, and XIII) and their cofactors (factors VIII, V, and HMWK) (Figure 1-2). All of the involved enzymes except factor XIII belong to a class known as serine proteases, most of which have substrate specificity. Factor XIII is a transpeptidase, which introduces peptide bonds into fibrin.

Blood coagulation is initiated in vitro by contact with a syringe or test tube. However, in vivo, activation is usually initiated by changes in endothelial cells or exposure of subendothelial components such as collagen. In either case, the series of reactions by which this activation culminates in the formation of fibrin is referred to as the *intrinsic pathway*. This is a relatively slow process.

More specifically, whenever blood comes in contact with negatively charged surfaces either in vitro or in vivo, the molecular configuration of factor XII is changed; and in concert with HMWK and prekallikrein, which it converts to kallikrein, it becomes an active serine protease (XII_a). This activated enzyme is then able to bring about a similar change in factor XI, a reaction also requiring the presence of HMWK. All of these reactions can be grouped together and considered to represent the process of contact activation. The factors involved in contact activation are present in very low concentrations in plasma.

The role of factor XII has always been somewhat of a paradox, as have the roles of prekallikrein and HMWK, because they appear to be essential for the initiation of clotting in vitro, but are not necessary for in vivo hemostasis. Persons who lack these factors do not suffer from hemorrhagic symptoms, even though patients lacking the related contact factor XI do bleed. Obviously, some other way must exist for factor XI to become activated in vivo. It has been shown that activated platelets may provide such a stimulus and that this reaction requires kallikrein. Since factor XII has other known actions, one of which is the activation of the fibrinolytic system, some patients who lack this factor have been found to suffer from thromboses because of defective fibrinolysis rather than hemorrhagic problems.

Activated factor XI is able to convert factor IX to its active serine protease form (IX_a). This reaction requires the presence of calcium, as do all of the remaining reactions except the action of thrombin (II_a) on fibrinogen (I). Factor IX is present in low concentration and is activated by a complex, two-stage reaction, which is apparently very slow, taking even a longer time than the initial contact reactions.

Activated factor IX (IX_a) requires cofactor VIII, Ca^{++}, and the phospholipid surface provided by activated platelets (PF_3) to bring about the activation of factor X. The role of the coagulant portion of the factor VIII molecule (VIII : C) in this reaction has not been totally defined, but it seems likely that it acts as a regulatory protein, enhancing the rate of factor X activation and that its ability to do this is greatly enhanced by the action on it of trace amounts of thrombin. The platelet phospholipid seems to act both to increase the local concentration of reactants by binding them to the lipid surface and also by inducing conformational changes in the protein components.

Factor X may also be converted to its active serine protease form (X_a) by a complex of tissue factor (thromboplastin, factor III), activated factor VII (VII_a) and Ca^{++}. The lipid surface required for this reaction is supplied by tissue factor, which is a lipoprotein complex. At least part of the factor VII molecules appear to circulate in an activated state, but are unable to act on factor X until a complex is formed with the protein moiety of tissue factor. Factor VII_a is also known to interact with factors XII_a and IX_a. The coagulation process initiated by the formation of the tissue factor–VII_a complex is referred to as the *extrinsic pathway* and all necessary components are present in plasma except the initiator, tissue factor, which becomes readily available from injured cells. Sequential reactions within this pathway occur rapidly.

The conversion of prothrombin (II) to thrombin (II_a) can occur via either the intrinsic or extrinsic pathway as a result of the proteolytic action of factor X_a in the presence of cofactor V, Ca^{++}, and a phospholipid surface. Factor V, especially when activated by thrombin, greatly accelerates this reaction but has no activity of its own. Phospholipid and Ca^{++} increase the rate of thrombin formation 30 to 100 fold. The same amount of thrombin that is produced in 1 minute with the normal physiologic amounts of factor X_a, Ca^{++}, factor V, and phospholipid would require 1 to 2 weeks to be produced by factor X_a alone. Factor X is present in much greater concentration than most of the factors that interact earlier in the coagulation process, and the concentration of prothrombin (II) is 10 times that of factor X. Many interactions appear to exist between the intrinsic and extrinsic pathways, so that as one becomes activated the other also participates in the coagulation process. It does not, however, appear that one can substitute for the other.

Human plasma is capable of generating large amounts of thrombin (130 to 160 clotting units/ml). During physiologic activation of the clotting process, however, thrombin concentrations do not exceed 10 clotting units/ml despite the consumption of almost all of the prothrombin content of plasma. This is due to the inactivation of thrombin by antithrombin, its conversion to prethrombin I, which is inactive, and its incorporation into the fibrin clot. Other control mechanisms probably operate at earlier steps in the coagulation process to ensure that the yield of thrombin reflects the size of the initial stimulus.

The interaction of thrombin (II_a) with fibrinogen (I) to form fibrin monomers initiates the final phase of blood coagulation. Fibrinogen is a rod-shaped protein (MW 340,000) composed of two monomeric units, each containing alpha, beta, and gamma chains, and is present in large amounts in plasma. The first stage of this reaction is the removal of the small A peptides from both of the alpha chains, allowing end-to-end association of molecules. This is followed by the removal of B peptides from the beta chains and lateral association of the molecules. The peptides make up only about 3% of the fibrinogen by weight, and the remaining portion of each molecule is referred to as a fibrin monomer. The fibrin polymers formed from these monomers are susceptible to the action of proteolytic enzymes, but thrombin is also able to activate factor XIII, which in its activated form, brings about cross linking and formation of an insoluble fibrin clot (Figure 1-3). Calcium is required for thrombin's activation of factor XIII but not for its proteolytic action on fibrinogen. Thrombin is a potent enzyme and has other significant actions. It is able to cause platelet aggregation and to convert factors VIII and V to their more active forms, both of which constitute positive feed-back mechanisms that accelerate clotting.

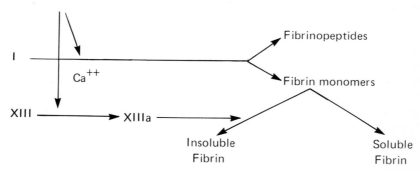

Figure 1-3. Fibrin polymerization reaction showing activation of factor XIII, which allows formation of insoluble fibrin.

Kinetics of Coagulation

Both intrinsic and extrinsic pathways require the interaction of multiple plasma-clotting factors. In either pathway, lack of a single factor will delay the conversion of factor II (prothrombin) to factor II_a (thrombin), which is the central event. In addition to clotting factors, the intrinsic system requires platelet phospholipid and the extrinsic system requires tissue thromboplastin, which contains a lipid component. Clotting factors normally are present in relative excess; platelet phospholipid appears to be the limiting factor in determining the rate of the reactions of the intrinsic pathway. Approximately 10 to 20% of the total number of platelets actually participate in the formation of thrombin, furnishing phospholipid surfaces and clotting factors for two of the central clotting reactions. The importance of platelets lies in the fact that they not only store and secrete various coagulation proteins but also bind coagulation enzymes to their surfaces, where these enzymes are protected from inactivation and where reactions among them can take place. If phospholipid is added in excess, the speed of clotting can be greatly accelerated; whereas increases in the levels of coagulation factors have little accelerating effect.

Coagulation, once initiated by either the intrinsic or extrinsic pathway, tends to accelerate. This process is, however, self-limiting and reaches a steady state. Thrombin activity is eventually neutralized and the plasminogen-plasmin system is activated which can bring about destruction of unneeded fibrin.

FIBRINOLYTIC SYSTEM

Fortunately, the formation of fibrin is not often permanent, and the body has many ways of disposing of unneeded fibrin. One is the enzymatic destruction of fibrin polymers into fragments that are no longer able to form a coherent fibrin network. This process of fibrinolysis is a normal physiologic mechanism; however, it may be exaggerated or depressed.

Plasminogen, a beta globulin with a molecular weight of about 90,000, which is present in plasma, can be converted into an active enzyme, plasmin, by activator substances. Activator substances are present in tissues, plasma, and blood vessel walls, and their secretion from vessels can be stimulated by such things as physical exercise, anxiety, and local ischemia. Such substances appear to be more abundant in veins than in arteries, and in organs with high metabolic activity such as the myocardium, brain, renal medulla, and endocrine glands.

A striking similarity exists between the blood coagulation system and the fibrinolytic system (Figure 1-4). The active enzymes (thrombin and plasmin) originate from precursors (prothrombin and plasminogen), which are both present in plasma. Thrombin and plasmin can each be formed by two different pathways of activation. One pathway is dependent entirely on humoral (intrinsic) factors present in plasma; the other is initiated by locally released tissue (extrinsic) factors. Both pathways have active inhibitors (antithrombin, antiplasmin).

When a fibrin clot forms, between 20 and 30% of the plasminogen content of plasma is trapped in the clot. Activators from plasma, tissues, or capillaries adsorb onto or diffuse into the clot and activate the plasminogen to plasmin. These reactions are usually localized, and should they occur in the circulating blood, are rapidly neutralized by inhibitors present in plasma. Thus, physiologic fibrinolysis can be accomplished locally without significant products of circulating fibrinolytic activity (Figure 1-5).

The lysis of fibrin clots by plasmin results in the formation of several degradation products. Similar fragments are formed from fibrinogen when the plasminogen activators, urokinase and streptokinase, are administered therapeutically. These

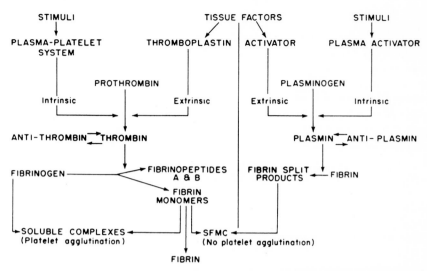

Figure 1-4.   Comparison of the plasminogen-plasmin system to the blood clotting system. (From Thal AP, et al: Shock, A Physiological Basis for Treatment. Chicago, Year Book Medical Publishers, Copyright © 1971. Used by permission.)

fibrinogen-fibrin degradation products (FDP) are partially digested fragments of fibrinogen or fibrin that have antigenic determinants in common with fibrinogen (Figure 1-6). They are referred to by the letters X, Y, D, and E. Fragment X, which is formed first by the splitting off of three small fragments, (A, B, and C) is the largest. It is slowly clottable and has a significant anticoagulant effect. Fragment Y is formed by the cleavage of fragment D from fragment X, and is eventually degraded to a molecule each of fragments D and E. Fragments D and E do not have significant anticoagulant activity. Under normal conditions, FDP are found in serum in minute

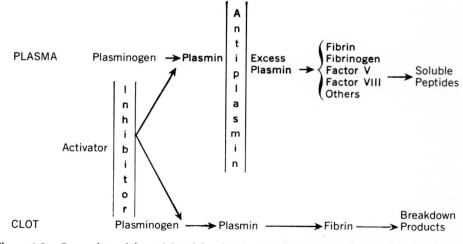

Figure 1-5.   Comparison of the activity of the plasminogen-plasmin system in plasma and in the clot.

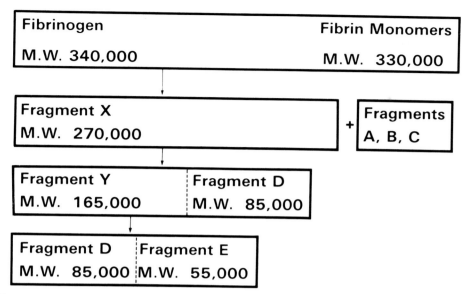

Figure 1-6.   Fibrinogen-fibrin degradation products (FDP) formed by the action of plasmin on fibrinogen or fibrin monomers.

quantities, undetectable by the usual tests; but they may be increased in serum samples of many hospitalized patients.

When small amounts of thrombin are formed in vivo, producing minimal fibrin polymer production, fibrin monomers may complex with intact fibrinogen molecules. If some intravascular fibrin is formed and fibrinolysis occurs, complexes may also be formed between the larger fibrin fragments, fibrin monomers and fibrinogen molecules. These soluble complexes are physiologically protective in preventing the further polymerization of fibrin monomers and are called soluble fibrin monomer complexes (SFMC) (Figure 1-7). They may be slowly clottable or nonclottable and so may be present in plasma or serum or both.

NATURAL INHIBITORS OF COAGULATION AND FIBRINOLYSIS

Efficient protective mechanisms limit the hemostatic process. These include the effects of blood flow in preventing the concentration of procoagulants at a given place and the clearance of activated coagulation factors from the circulation by the liver and the reticuloendothelial system. Fibrin has a nonspecific adsorbing action on thrombin. Also, a variety of substances that are present in normal blood oppose the action of thrombin and the other serine proteases that become activated during coagulation.

Proteins C and S of plasma have recently been shown to be possible modulators of blood coagulation. Protein C is a serine protease that when activated by thrombin, can degrade factors V and VIII:C, and protein S apparently serves as a cofactor for these reactions. Protein C is a vitamin K-dependent factor.

Antithrombin III has been shown to be the most effective inhibitor of serine proteases and is known to form 1:1 stoichiometric complexes with thrombin and the

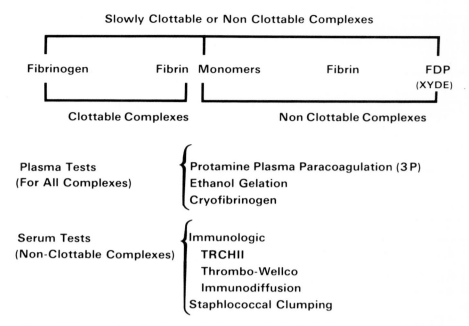

Figure 1-7. Formation of and methods of testing for soluble fibrin monomer complexes.

activated forms of factors XII, XI, IX, X, and kallikrein in slow one-step reactions that render them inactive (Figure 1-8). Its interaction with factor VII, which appears to circulate in its active form, is less clear. An arginine residue of AT III is the site that reacts with the serine sites of the activated clotting proteins. AT III is also a potent antiplasmin, and it inactivates some of the activated complement components; however, its most important action appears to be its inhibition of thrombin. Because the quantity of AT III in plasma is ten times that of factor X, but is about equal to the quantity of prothrombin, a measurable depletion of AT III requires massive activation of factor X but only minor activation of prothrombin. It has been estimated by the use of model equations that the free thrombin level approximately doubles in a reaction mixture if the AT III level falls to 70% and quadruples if it falls to 50%.

$$\boxed{\text{AT III} + \text{II}_a} \longrightarrow \boxed{\text{AT III-II}_a \text{ Complex}}$$

$(\text{XII}_a, \text{XI}_a, \text{IX}_a, \text{X}_a)$ formed slowly

Although six different antithrombins have been described in the literature, only antithrombin III has proved to be of clinical significance. Its stability in whole blood, plasma, or serum is remarkable, with no loss occurring with up to 4 weeks of storage at 4° C. Levels of AT III in serum are about 30 to 40% lower than in plasma, which indicates that AT III is more than adequate to inhibit the activated serine proteases formed during in vitro clotting. The neutralization of serine proteases by AT III has been shown to be dramatically accelerated by heparin; hence, it is sometimes referred to as heparin cofactor (previously named antithrombin II). Heparin molecules bind to lysine residues on the AT III molecules and produce conformational changes

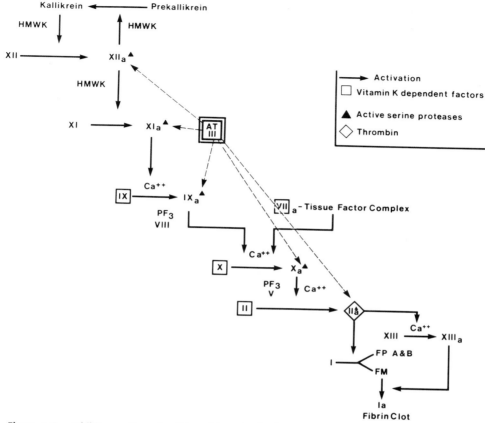

Figure 1-8. Inhibitory action of antithrombin III by the formation of complexes with the active serine protease forms of factors XII, XI, IX, X, and II.

that render their reactive arginine sites more accessible for neutralization of the active sites of the protease enzymes.

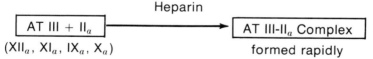

Knowledge of this interaction is of importance in understanding the use of heparin as an anticoagulant. Since either heparin or AT III may be rate limiting, adequate concentrations of both must be present to produce an anticoagulant effect. Tissue mast cells, which contain heparin, are sometimes located near vascular surfaces, and it is possible that a physiologic anticoagulant effect may be produced if they are stimulated to produce heparin locally, which can then interact with circulating AT III.

Other inhibitors, such as α-1-antitrypsin and α-2-macroglobulin also neutralize the activity of the proteolytic enzymes of the coagulation system, but they do not seem to play major roles in thrombin modulation. Alpha-2-macroglobulin and C1 esterase do, however, function in regulating the early steps in the contact phase of coagulation.

Dissolution of fibrin or fibrinogenolysis is also checked or retarded by natural inhibitors, which may inhibit the conversion of plasminogen to plasmin or act upon plasmin already formed. At least five inhibitors have been shown to inhibit plasmin in purified systems in vitro. Such reactions are apparently stoichiometric (1:1). Alpha-2-antiplasmin is considered to be the most important of these inhibitors even though it is present in a much lower molar concentration than α-1-antitrypsin, α-2-macroglobulin, C1 esterase, and AT III. This is because of its great affinity for plasmin. In addition to these inhibitors in plasma, tissue and platelets also contain inhibitors of fibrinolysis.

References

Aoki N: Natural inhibitors of fibrinolysis. Prog Cardiovasc Dis 21:267, 1979.

Bowie EJW: Thrombosis and atherosclerosis: Willebrand factor and platelets. Primary Cardiol 7:51, 1981.

Caen JP, Cronberg S., and Jubisz P: Platelets: Physiology and Pathology. New York, Stratton Intercontinental Book Corp, 1977.

Chesterman CN: The fibrinolytic system and haemostasis. Thromb Diath Haemorrh 34:368, 1975.

Esnouf MP: Biochemistry of blood coagulation. Br Med Bull 33:213, 1977.

Henry RL: Platelet function. Semin Thromb Hemostas 4:93, 1977.

Kaplan AP, Meier HL, and Mandle RJ Jr: The role of Hageman factor, prekallikrein and high molecular weight kininogen in the generation of bradykinin and the initiation of coagulation and fibrinolysis. Monogr Allergy 12:120, 1977.

Kernoff PBA, and McNicol GP: Normal and abnormal fibrinolysis. Br Med Bull 33:239, 1977.

Murano G: A basic outline of blood coagulation. Semin Thromb Hemostas 6:140, 1980.

Rosenberg RD: Chemistry of the hemostatic mechanism and its relationship to the action of heparin. Fed Proc 36:10, 1977.

Rosenberg RD: Hemorrhagic Disorders I. Protein interactions in the clotting mechanism. In Hematology. Edited by WS Beck. Cambridge, MIT Press, 1977.

Seegers WH: Antithrombin-III: function and assay. Lab Manag 9:23, 1981.

Triplett DA, et al: Platelet Function: Laboratory Evaluation and Clinical Application. Chicago, ASCP, 1978.

Walsh PN: Platelets and coagulation proteins. Fed Proc 40:2086, 1981.

Wintrobe MM, et al: Clinical Hematology, 8th Ed. Philadelphia, Lea & Febiger, 1982.

CHAPTER *2*

Disorders of Hemostasis and Thrombosis

VASCULAR ABNORMALITIES

Disorders of blood vessels may be inherited or acquired, localized or generalized, and may result in abnormal bleeding or thrombosis. They thus constitute a wide variety of conditions.

Clinically, the diagnosis of such problems depends primarily on careful personal and family histories and on a complete physical examination, including special emphasis on examination of the skin and mucous membranes. Venography, arteriography, and endoscopy have made it possible to visualize some of the larger and less accessible vascular lesions. Microtechniques have also provided a means for studying endothelium in vivo, and there are in vitro techniques for culturing endothelial cells. Such procedures have contributed to an understanding of endothelial physiology and pathophysiology.

The role of the clinical laboratory in the diagnosis of vascular disorders remains peripheral, and in most instances, all hemostatic tests give normal values. But because many patients with thrombohemorrhagic disorders that are due to vascular abnormalities will be referred to the laboratory for diagnostic studies, it is important to be informed about them. Again, the recent emphasis on the important role of blood vessels themselves in the etiology of thrombotic problems has drawn special attention to this aspect of the hemostatic mechanism.

The most common laboratory features of hemorrhagic vascular disorders are the following: an abnormal tourniquet test, an abnormal bleeding time (particularly an abnormal aspirin tolerance test), and the demonstration of normal numbers and function of platelets. Vascular and platelet function are closely related, and in some situations, abnormalities in both may occur simultaneously. Presently utilized platelet function tests may not detect mild abnormalities, so some conditions that are thought to be related primarily to vascular abnormalities may, in reality, represent mild platelet function disorders.

Vascular disorders may be classified as follows:
A. Defects of structure (primarily inherited)
   1. Hereditary hemorrhagic telangiectasia and other angiodysplasias.
   2. Connective tissue dysplasias.

17

    3. Vascular purpura.
  B. Defects of strength, permeability, and surface (primarily acquired)
    1. "Easy bruisability."
    2. Increased vascular fragility.
    3. Senile or steroid purpura.
    4. Petechiae associated with increased intracapillary pressure.
    5. Autoimmune disorders associated with thrombohemorrhagic phenomena.
    6. Drug toxicity.
    7. Purpura associated with systemic disease.
    8. Local changes in vessels.
  C. Psychogenic purpura

Defects of Structure
Hereditary Hemorrhagic Telangiectasia

Hereditary hemorrhagic telangiectasia (HHT) is the most common hereditary vascular disorder leading to a hemorrhagic diathesis. The disorder is inherited as an autosomal dominant, but the lesions do not usually become prominent until the third decade of life or later. Epistaxis, which is the hallmark of the disorder, may begin in early childhood and usually decreases with age. Most studies have shown that the localized lesions develop because elastic fibers are missing in vascular walls. The lesions are made up of coiled dilated capillaries and venules from which bleeding can easily occur if the lesions are located close to a surface. These lesions may be pinpoint, nodular, or spider-like, and they are seen primarily on skin and mucous membranes (palmar surfaces of fingers and hands, fingernails, nasal septum, lips, and tongue). Since these abnormalities may be generalized throughout the body, they can also cause gastrointestinal and genitourinary hemorrhage, hemoptysis, and heavy menses. Approximately 20% of patients develop arteriovenous (A-V) fistulas of the lungs, and there is also a high incidence of Laennec's type cirrhosis. The bleeding time is usually normal and the tourniquet test may be normal or abnormal. Abnormal platelet function tests have been reported in some patients with the syndrome. Although there is usually no significant abnormality in blood coagulation, it has recently been reported that many patients have an associated disseminated intravascular coagulation-type syndrome, which is most often present in chronic form but periodically can become acute.

Giant cavernous hemangiomata are similar to the lesions of HHT, but are much larger and are usually present at birth. They are associated with recurrent acute thrombosis and disseminated intravascular coagulation (DIC), the so-called Kasabach-Merritt syndrome. Many other angiodysplastic syndromes of the gastrointestinal tract have been described. These may be hereditary or degenerative. Such lesions have been seen in association with von Willebrand's disease and aortic stenosis.

Treatment involves local obliteration of bleeding lesions, if possible. When disseminated intravascular coagulation is present, heparin may be useful. When there is extensive involvement of the gastrointestinal tract and nasal mucosa, blood loss may become excessive, and the patient often requires repeated transfusions and continuous iron therapy.

Connective Tissue Dysplasias

These rare hereditary conditions include the Ehlers-Danlos syndrome, Marfan's syndrome, and osteogenesis imperfecta, which are inherited as autosomal dominants, and pseudoxanthoma elasticum and homocystinuria, which have autosomal recessive inheritance. The basic pathology appears to be a combination of variable defects in the structure of collagen (which normally supports blood vessels) and abnormalities in elastic fibers. A defect in fibronectin (an adhesive glycoprotein that cross links to collagen) has been described in one kindred with Ehlers-Danlos syndrome. Easy bruisability is common to all of these conditions, but more significant problems such as gingival bleeding, epistaxis, gastrointestinal bleeding, hemoptysis, and intraarticular bleeding may also occur. Marfan's syndrome is the least characterized clinically by a hemorrhagic diathesis. Patients with pseudoxanthoma elasticum have the most severe bleeding problems as well as a predisposition to thrombosis. Cardiovascular abnormalities are also commonly seen in these conditions. Treatment is not very successful.

Common laboratory abnormalities include a positive tourniquet test, prolonged bleeding time, and in some instances, associated platelet functional defects that may be related to abnormalities in fibronectin.

Vascular Purpura

Vascular purpura is a general designation that has been used to refer to a variety of conditions that are characterized by a prolonged bleeding time and a normal platelet count. Bleeding is usually mild to moderate and is manifested primarily by easy bruising and mucous membrane bleeding. When no specific evidence of associated platelet dysfunction and no deficiency of plasma coagulation factors exist, it is assumed that the defect lies in the blood vascular system, although there is no absolute proof of this. Such a diagnosis depends on the demonstration of a prolonged bleeding time in a patient in whom the reactions to all other hemostatic tests are normal. It is actually a diagnosis by exclusion. The tourniquet test also occasionally shows abnormality, but this finding is not as characteristic as the prolongation of the bleeding time. The clinical severity of bleeding problems fluctuates considerably in patients with vascular purpura; the bleeding time may vary from time to time and may show significant prolongation when the subject has taken aspirin or other nonsteroidal, anti-inflammatory drugs. If vascular purpura is suspected and the bleeding time at the patient's initial examination is found to be within the normal limits, the test should be repeated on several occasions. Since most of these patients have not been studied with a variety of platelet function tests, it is possible that many of them actually suffer from minor abnormalities of platelet function rather than from vascular abnormalities. Corticosteroids have been found useful in therapy, especially when used prophylactically prior to dental extractions.

Characteristic findings in vascular purpura are the following:
1. Normal platelet numbers and morphology.
2. Increased bleeding time.

3. Normal or abnormal reaction to the tourniquet test.
4. Normal clot retraction.
5. Possible abnormalities in platelet retention in glass bead columns, aggregation, or platelet-factor-3 availability.
6. Normal activated partial thromboplastin time and prothrombin time.

Defects of Strength, Permeability, and Surface

Easy Bruisability

This term is used to describe an increased tendency to formation of superficial ecchymoses without abnormalities demonstrable by hemostatic tests. The condition appears more often in females than in males, probably because of the ineffective support of vascular structures by the more abundant subcutaneous fatty tissue in females. Bruises occur most often on the thighs and upper arms where the greatest quantity of fat is present. It has been suggested that such easy bruisability may be associated with hypothyroidism in some cases. The bleeding time is usually normal. The platelets are normal in number and morphology. It is possible that variable abnormalities may be demonstrated in platelet function. The most common abnormalities we have seen are a slight prolongation of the template bleeding time and a decrease in the retention of platelets in glass bead columns. Coagulation studies are normal.

Increased Vascular Fragility

Another vague term, increased vascular fragility, may be applied to designate a tendency to increased bruising and bleeding, with the only positive finding being that of a positive tourniquet test. The platelets are normal morphologically and in number, but most patients have not been tested extensively for abnormalities of platelet function. Coagulation studies are normal.

Senile or Steroid Purpura

The hemorrhagic lesions seen in elderly persons occur primarily on the extensor surfaces of the forearms and backs of the hands. The hemorrhages are characteristically superficial, dark purple, and of variable size, usually about 1 to 10 mm in diameter. They appear to result from extravasation of blood in response to minor trauma and may be easily produced by applying blunt, shearing stress to the skin. They resorb slowly and leave a considerable amount of blood pigment in the skin. The defect lies in degenerative changes in the skin that result in a lack of elasticity of the connective tissues around the superficial vessels. Corticosteroids produce the same type of skin changes. Reactions to all the hemostatic tests are normal, and the patients do not show abnormal bleeding tendencies elsewhere on the body.

Petechiae Associated with Increased Intracapillary Pressure

In situations in which there is a sudden local increase in the pressure within capillaries, a fine petechial rash may develop. The two most common conditions producing this are convulsive seizures and extreme prolonged coughing paroxysms such as those that occur with whooping cough. The petechiae usually appear on the head and neck and disappear rapidly. Results of hemostatic tests are all normal.

Autoimmune Disorders Associated with Thrombohemorrhagic Phenomena

Immunologic diseases associated with circulating antibodies and immune complexes can result in a variety of conditions in which vasculitis occurs with thrombosis and/or hemorrhage. In disorders such as allergic purpura (Henoch-Schönlein) and polyarteritis an antibody is directed specifically against endothelium. Allergic purpura occurs most often in children and is characterized by a symmetrical, diffuse, petechial or purpuric rash, usually confined to the lower extremities and buttocks, but occasionally involving the upper extremities.

Many more autoimmune-type disorders exist in which antibodies and immune complexes damage not only endothelium but other cellular systems and in which damage also occurs to perivascular tissues. Many infectious agents (bacteria, rickettsia, viruses, and mycoplasma) produce vasculitis with thrombohemorrhagic manifestations in this way. Similar disorders include collagen-vascular disease (e.g., systemic lupus erythematosis), drug reactions, and some lymphoreticular syndromes.

Drug Toxicity

The hemorrhagic rashes that occur with drug toxicity may resemble those seen in allergic purpura but may be more severe, actually advancing to skin necrosis and gangrene. Drugs induce vasculitis in a variety of ways: direct effect on the vessel wall, the development of specific antivessel antibodies, and the development of circulating immune complexes. Commonly used drugs that have been associated with such toxicity are listed in Table 2-1. Coumadin can produce severe hemorrhagic

TABLE 2-1.   Common Drugs Causing Vasculitis

Allopurinol	Estrogens	Methyldopa
Arsenicals	Furosemide	Piperazine
Aspirin	Gold Salts	Quinidine
Chloramphenicol	Indomethacin	Quinine
Chlorpropamide	Iodine	Reserpine
Coumadin [sodium warfarin]	Isoniazid	Sulfonamides
Digoxin	Meprobamate	Tolbutamide

Bick RL: Vascular disorders associated with Thrombohemorrhagic Phenomena. Semin Thromb Hemostas 5:180, 1979.

vasculitis with skin infarction and associated intravascular coagulation. In drug-related problems, the bleeding time and platelet count are usually normal, but the reaction to the tourniquet test may be positive. Coagulation tests are normal unless there is associated DIC.

Manifestations of Systemic Disease

Acute infections, diabetes, uremia, malignant paraprotein disorders, scurvy, and hypothyroidism are often accompanied by generalized or local changes in blood vessels. Hemorrhagic problems are usually not of great importance, but increased fragility and permeability of the vessels may cause generalized petechiae or purpura, retinal hemorrhages, and epistaxis. Thromboses are also frequent complications, particularly in diabetes and malignant hypertension. Downstream capillary stasis, which occurs after deep venous thromboses, may lead to chronic purpura in the lower extremities.

Numerous hemorrhagic and thrombotic problems are seen with malignant para-protein disorders and may be related to increased levels of a paraprotein that fixes complement to vessels, hyperviscosity, cryoglobulinemia, thrombocytopenia and associated amyloidosis. In these kinds of disorders, the reaction to the tourniquet test is occasionally positive.

Patients with renal failure often have moderately reduced platelet counts and decreased availability of platelet factor 3. Diminished platelet retention and aggregation have also been demonstrated. Platelet function is usually improved by dialysis, often in parallel with improvement in the bleeding tendency. A selective factor X deficiency has been reported in patients with amyloidosis, and the thrombin time, prothrombin time, and activated partial thromboplastin time may all be prolonged due to the interference of paraproteins in fibrin polymerization.

Local Changes in Vessels

In many cases, thrombohemorrhagic phenomena are related to localized changes in the vessels themselves. Inflammation causes dilatation of vessels and increased permeability. Infectious agents may damage vessels through direct infiltration or by the action of toxins. Ulceration and trauma may produce disruption or destruction of vessel walls. Hemorrhage into tumors is common because of rapid growth and necrosis. The formation of ulcerated plaques in atherosclerotic vessels may result in thrombus formation, dissection, and rupture.

Psychogenic Purpuras

The literature includes reports of a diverse group of patients, mainly women with significant emotional disorders, who have had cutaneous bruising or bleeding through apparently intact skin. They also have a wide variety of associated systemic symptoms. Descriptive diagnoses have included autoerythrocyte sensitization, DNA sensitization, factitial purpura, and the religious stigmata. Hemostatic tests give normal results, but the intracutaneous injection of erythrocyte stroma, whole blood, or washed red cells is usually reported to evoke typical inflammatory hemorrhagic lesions. The pathogenesis is unclear but includes the possibility of a conversion reaction, some type of immunologic disorder, or a somatic response to psychologic problems.

References

Bick RL: Vascular disorders associated with thrombo-hemorrhagic phenomena. Semin Thromb Hemostas 5:167, 1979.

Nydegger UE, Miescher UE: Bleeding due to vascular disorders. Semin Hematol 17:178, 1980.

Ratnoff OD: The psychogenic purpuras: a review of autoerythrocyte sensitization, autosensitization to DNA, "hysterical" and factitial bleeding, and the religious stigmata. Semin Hematol 17:192, 1980.

Stepfens WE: Hemodynamics and the Blood Vessel Wall. Springfield, Charles C Thomas, 1979.

PLATELET ABNORMALITIES

Since platelets act both mechanically and as part of the coagulation mechanism, it is necessary not only that they be present in adequate numbers, but also that they function properly. It is impossible to evaluate functional capacity from the ordinary light microscopic examination of platelets, although abnormally functioning platelets may sometimes be bizarre in appearance. Electron microscopy has proved to be helpful in this area of investigation. At the present time, functional evaluation is dependent primarily on such tests as the bleeding time, clot retraction, platelet factor 3 availability, platelet aggregation, and platelet retention in glass bead columns.

Platelet abnormalities may be classified as follows:

A. Quantitative platelet disorders
    1. Thrombocytopenia.
    2. Thrombocytosis.
B. Qualitative platelet disorders
    1. Defects of platelet adhesiveness
      a. Diminished adhesiveness (e.g. von Willebrand's disease, Bernard-Soulier syndrome).
    2. Defects of platelet aggregation
      a. Diminished primary aggregation (e.g., thrombasthenia).
      b. Abnormal secondary aggregation and release reaction (storage pool disease, "aspirin-like" defect, drug-related abnormalities).
      c. Spontaneous aggregation.
    3. Combined defects and defects of platelet interaction.

Quantitative Platelet Disorders

Quantitative platelet disorders may be related to both hemorrhagic and thrombotic abnormalities. Thrombocytopenia is primarily related to bleeding problems, but increased platelet numbers can result in both hemorrhage and thrombosis.

Thrombocytopenia

Thrombocytopenia may be due to: (a) production defects; (b) distributional defects; (c) dilutional loss; and (d) abnormal destruction. The diseases in which production is the problem are primarily those in which an abnormality in the bone marrow results in a reduction in the number of megakaryocytes available to produce platelets. A bone marrow examination usually reveals a decrease or absence of megakaryocytes and, in some instances, specific abnormalities to account for the decrease such as aplasia or hypoplasia, leukemia, lymphoma, preleukemia, multiple myeloma, myelofibrosis, or metastatic carcinoma. In megaloblastic anemias due to vitamin B_{12} or folic acid deficiency, moderate thrombocytopenia is common and is associated with maturation abnormalities in megakaryocytes similar to those seen in the red cell series. Familial thrombocytopenia is also usually associated with abnormal megakaryopoiesis.

Splenomegaly produces a distributional defect by enlarging the splenic platelet pool, and this usually results in variable degrees of thrombocytopenia. In some myeloproliferative disorders, the rate of production may be increased enough to result in thrombocytosis rather than thrombocytopenia despite massive splenic enlargement.

When acute hemorrhage is treated with massive transfusions of platelet-poor blood, circulating platelets are decreased because of a delay in replacement, and a temporary dilutional thrombocytopenia is the result. Dilutional thrombocytopenia and increased destruction both occur with the extracorporeal circulation of blood during cardiopulmonary bypass.

Abnormal destruction of platelets may occur due to consumption in disseminated intravascular coagulation (DIC) and in patients with giant hemangiomas and thrombotic thrombocytopenia purpura. Infectious agents may damage platelets directly or be associated with the development of antibodies that produce autoimmune destruction. Drug-related thrombocytopenias are primarily autoimmune but may be due to a direct toxic effect of a drug on the bone marrow. The most common drug-related autoimmune thrombocytopenia is that due to quinidine or quinine in which an antibody is formed to a drug-protein complex. Platelets provide a surface to which this antigen antibody complex can adhere and are destroyed in the process.

The prototype of autoimmune thrombocytopenia is the syndrome called idiopathic thrombocytopenic purpura (ITP), which may be acute or chronic. Since tests for platelet antibodies are technically difficult and are still unstandardized, this diagnosis is frequently made without laboratory confirmation of the presence of antibodies. The pathophysiologic mechanism involved is the attachment of antibodies to the surfaces of platelets, which then allows their rapid clearance from the circulation by splenic or liver macrophages.

Neonatal thrombocytopenias may be associated with sepsis, due to the transfer of maternal platelet autoantibodies or to the formation by a mother who lacks the PLA-1 antigen of an isoimmune antibody to the PLA-1 antigen of the fetus (as in erythroblastosis fetalis). Only 1 to 2% of the population lacks the PLA-1 antigen, so the last situation is not common; but a related problem is the development of post-transfusion purpura in PLA-1 negative subjects.

In all of these situations, the low platelet count is the most significant finding. The lack of platelets may also result in abnormalities in the bleeding time, clot retraction, and other platelet function tests, although these tests are usually of no help in making a specific diagnosis or in monitoring therapy. It may be somewhat dangerous to do the bleeding time test in patients with severe thrombocytopenia because of the possibility of prolonged bleeding and hematoma formation at the site of the skin incision.

If the thrombocytopenia is secondary to a treatable disease, platelet counts may become higher when specific therapy is given. In the presence of increased auto-immune destruction, corticosteroids or splenectomy may be helpful. Some patients with thrombotic thrombocytopenic purpura have responded to a wide variety of therapeutic modalities, including corticosteroids, splenectomy, plasmapheresis, plasma infusions, antiplatelet drugs, and vincristine. Platelet transfusions are indicated in most acute bleeding situations that are due to a lack of platelets and in preparation of patients with such a problem for surgery except in those who have circulating autoantibodies. Repeated transfusions of platelets from random donors usually result in the development of platelet antibodies with an increasingly poor response to such therapy. Use of a single platelet donor, especially a family member, frequently results in a better yield and survival of infused platelets.

Characteristic findings in thrombocytopenia are the following:
1. Decreased platelet count.
2. Normal or prolonged bleeding time.
3. Frequently, abnormal reaction to the tourniquet test.
4. Abnormal clot retraction.
5. If patient's platelets are tested, the thromboplastin generation test may be abnormal. Other tests of platelet function require adjustment for platelet numbers.
6. Tests for platelet antibodies may be positive in autoimmune thrombocytopenia and in patients who have had multiple transfusions.
7. Special clot retraction and PF_3 tests for drug-related thrombocytopenia may be positive.
8. Normal prothrombin time and activated partial thromboplastin time.

Thrombocytosis

Patients with markedly elevated platelet counts may have repeated episodes of both thrombosis and spontaneous hemorrhage. Reactive thrombocytosis occurs commonly in association with malignancy, inflammation, hemolysis, the post-splenectomy state, and acute bleeding. In these conditions, platelet function tests are usually normal and the clinical problem minimal. When thrombocytosis occurs as a reflection of a myeloproliferative syndrome, platelets are frequently bizarre in appearance and have functional defects. Massive thrombosis may occur with associated bleeding. Such symptoms usually improve with treatment, which is aimed at lowering the platelet count. Characteristic findings in thrombocytosis include:
1. Increased numbers of platelets with bizarre morphology in myeloproliferative states.
2. Normal or prolonged bleeding time.
3. Usually, normal reaction to the tourniquet test.
4. Increased red cell fallout when clot retraction is tested.
5. If patient's platelets are tested, the thromboplastin generation test may be abnormal.
6. Variable abnormalities in platelet aggregation.
7. Possibly, abnormal platelet factor 3-availability test, even when the platelet count is adjusted to nearly normal.
8. Normal prothrombin time and activated partial thromboplastin time.

Qualitative Platelet Disorders

Qualitative disorders present a greater diagnostic problem than do the quantitative ones, and often it is extremely difficult to isolate them from vascular diseases. Both platelets and blood vessels are involved in the control of the bleeding time, and a test of the bleeding time is the screening procedure most often used in the study of both qualitative platelet disorders and vascular diseases. The patient with a long bleeding time and normal platelet count could easily have either abnormally functioning platelets or vascular disease or both. The findings reported by different investigators have varied widely, and there are probably many mixed and ill-defined forms that do not fit any classification. Table 2-2 gives detailed differential information about the major inherited qualitative disorders of platelets.

The disorders in a group of 70 patients with prolonged bleeding times and normal platelet counts were diagnosed as follows:

von Willebrand's disease	30
Isolated prolonged bleeding time (vascular purpura?)	19
Thrombasthenia	11
Thrombocytopathy with abnormal platelet morphology	5
Thrombocytopathy with normal platelet morphology	5

Defects of Platelet Adhesiveness

von Willebrand's disease (Table 2-2), which is an extrinsic defect of adhesion, may be the most common genetic hemorrhagic defect. It was first described in patients from the Aland Islands near Finland in 1926. Although the platelet counts were normal in these patients, their platelet function and blood vessels were thought to be abnormal to account for prolongation of their bleeding times. Their bleeding was primarily nasal, gingival, subcutaneous, and from the uterine endometrium; although gastrointestinal bleeding, hemarthroses, and excessive blood loss after tooth extraction and tonsillectomy were also described. Later, it was found that many of the affected patients also had moderately decreased levels of factor VIII coagulant activity (VIII:C less than 40%) and also decreased platelet adhesiveness in vivo and vitro. More recently, immunologic factor VIII (VIII R:Ag) has been found to be decreased or abnormal in patients with von Willebrand's disease. Most of them also lack the plasmatic activity that is necessary to induce platelet aggregation by ristocetin. This latter factor VIII-related activity is referred to as Willebrand factor (VIII R:WF).

The disease in both mild and severe forms occurs equally in both sexes and is usually of autosomal dominant inheritance, but of variable expressivity. The most severe cases are homozygotes with inheritance from both parents. The course of the disease fluctuates, and measurable levels of factor VIII coagulant activity and the degree of prolongation of the bleeding time have been shown to vary from time to time. The transfusion of plasma, even from hemophiliac patients, causes an increase in factor VIII coagulant activity considerably in excess of the amount expected. Cryoprecipitate preparations are also effective in producing such an effect, but the more purified concentrates of factor VIII are not. The fact that the bleeding time is transiently shortened by the administration of plasma and some plasma fractions is evidence that the platelets are not themselves intrinsically defective, but that they require a plasma factor to have normal in vivo adhesiveness. There is an exaggerated response of the bleeding time to aspirin ingestion, which would be expected because of the superimposition of the defect in platelet function caused by aspirin on the secondary defect already present in von Willebrand's disease.

TABLE 2-2. Major Inherited Disorders of Platelet Function

	Adhesion	Aggregation				Release (ADP, PF$_4$)	Clot Retraction	Basic Abnormality	Hemorrhagic Manifestations	Platelet Morphology Observed By Light Microscopy	Platelet Ultrastructure		Heredity
		Primary	Secondary	Ristocetin	Bovine F. VIII						TEM	SEM (Membrane Activation)	
Bernard-Soulier Syndrome	↓	N	N	Absent	Absent	N	N	Membrane abnormality (absent or decreased glycoprotein I complex)	Severe	Giant platelets (often great variation in size)	"Swiss cheese" platelets	Insufficient observations to comment	Autosomal recessive
Thrombasthenia	N	Absent	Absent	N	N	N	Absent or Poor	Membrane abnormality (absent or decreased glycoprotein IIb, IIIa; decreased actomyosin)	Variable but often severe (however, tendency to decrease with age)	Platelets isolated, not in clumps	N	Swollen, convoluted, stubby pseudopods	Autosomal recessive
Storage Pool Disease	N or ↓	N	↓	N	N	↓	N	Absent or decreased dense granule contents (storage pool ADP, ATP, Ca^{++}, serotonin)	Variable but usually mild	N	↓ or absent dense bodies	Flat forms	Hermansky-Pudlak—autosomal recessive. Storage pool deficiency—autosomal dominant
"Aspirin-like" Defects	N	N	↓	N	N	↓	N	Abnormalities in the release mechanism (heterogeneous group of disorders)	Usually mild	N	N	Disc forms, impaired pseudopods	Not clear; heterogeneous group of disorders
von Willebrand's Disease	↓	N	N	Absent	N	N	N	Abnormalities in the F. VIII/vWF protein. The defective protein may be incapable of acting as an intracellular bridge between platelets and the vessel wall (the platelets are intrinsically normal)	Variable (mild to severe)	N	N	Flat discs, atypical spread forms	Autosomal dominant with incomplete penetrance (many variants described)

N = normal. ↓ = decreased. It should be noted that the bleeding time is characteristically prolonged in all of these disorders. In general, no single test of platelet function or ultrastructure is pathognomonic of a particular disease state. Rather, several (or all) of the above mentioned abnormalities must be present.

Two basic types of patients have been identified. Type I patients have reduced levels or, in the most severe cases, almost complete absence of all of the normal factor VIII-related activities. Type II patients have milder forms of the disease and, rather than reduced amounts of factor VIII protein, have abnormal molecular forms of the protein which result in variable test results for the different factor VIII-related activities. In type IIA, there is an absence of the important larger molecular forms in both plasma and platelets. Such multimers are particularly important in supporting ristocetin aggregation. Type IIB patients have small molecular forms in their plasma but larger multimers in their platelets. This results in an unusual, heightened responsiveness in their platelets to ristocetin, despite decreased plasma factor VIII R:WF activity when measured by the ristocetin cofactor assay, which utilizes donor platelets. Abnormalities in the molecular forms of factor VIII can be demonstrated by crossed immunoelectrophoresis.

Several patients have been described in whom von Willebrand's disease has been acquired. These patients differ from those with the inherited disorder in that they fail to have the exaggerated rise in VIII:C after plasma infusion. The hemostatic defect may resolve if the condition with which it is associated achieves remission.

It is often a striking finding that there may be wide fluctuation in the bleeding time and factor VIII:C level in the same person on repeated testing. This was clearly demonstrated by a study in which factor VIII:C levels and modified Ivy bleeding-time tests were performed simultaneously 100 times on 27 clinically affected members of three families with von Willebrand's disease. Both values were abnormal on 53 occasions, only one or the other was abnormal on 36 occasions, and both were normal on 11 occasions. Because of the variable expressivity of this disease, the diagnosis may be particularly difficult, especially when family studies are not available. Also, tests may be "normalized" during pregnancy or when subjects take estrogens.

Laboratory findings in von Willebrand's disease include:
1. Normal platelet count and morphology.
2. Variably prolonged bleeding time (significantly increased by aspirin ingestion).
3. Normal or slight prolongation of the activated partial thromboplastin time, with a normal prothrombin time.
4. Normal clot retraction.
5. Normal platelet aggregation with all aggregating agents except ristocetin.
6. Normal or abnormal platelet factor 3-availability test.
7. Decreased platelet retention in glass bead columns (rarely normal).
8. Variable abnormalities in factor VIII-related activities.

The *Bernard-Soulier* syndrome is a rare, inherited, autosomal recessive disorder in which platelet adhesiveness is decreased and platelets do not aggregate at all when tested with ristocetin, even though all plasma factor VIII activities are normal (Table 2-2). The defect is due to a lack of a specific receptor protein (glycoprotein I) for factor VIII on the surface of the platelets. The platelets aggregate normally with ADP, adrenalin, and collagen. These patients usually have mild thrombocytopenia and megathrombocytes. Other related familial platelet syndromes have been described (e.g., Wiskott-Aldrich, May-Hegglin).

Platelet adhesiveness may also be decreased in patients with thrombasthenia and other intrinsic platelet disorders. Decreased adhesiveness has been described in afibrinogenemia and myeloproliferative syndromes. Adhesiveness is usually decreased in uremia. The administration of certain drugs (clofibrate, dextran, glyceryl guaiacolate, and dipyridamole) has been reported to decrease platelet adhesiveness. Aspirin does not appear to affect adhesiveness, and platelet retention in glass bead columns is normal in subjects taking aspirin.

Increased adhesiveness, which is frequently seen postoperatively when there is a pouring out of new platelets, may be associated with other hypercoagulable states. Increased adhesiveness has been shown to be associated with decreased platelet survival. Increased adhesiveness as measured by increased retention of platelets in glass bead columns can be demonstrated by utilizing special columns that contain larger beads than those used to demonstrate decreased adhesiveness.

Defects of Platelet Aggregation

Thrombasthenia, or Glanzmann's disease, is a defect of primary platelet aggregation (Table 2-2). It is a rare hereditary disorder with autosomal recessive inheritance. The homozygote has little tendency to spontaneous bleeding, with the exception of epistaxis and menorrhagia, but bleeding due to trauma or surgery is frequently excessive. There seems to be a tendency toward decreasing severity with age. In this condition, two major membrane glycoproteins (IIb and IIIa) are deficient, and as a result, aggregation is diminished, clot retraction decreased, and bleeding time prolonged, all of which are probably related to the inability of fibrinogen to bind to abnormal platelet surfaces and, in addition, to the absence or decrease of the membrane-linked contractile protein actomysin.

It is usually reported that heterozygous carriers of thrombasthenia are asymptomatic; but some of these persons have mild bleeding problems, particularly associated with trauma or surgery. We have studied the mother of one homozygote extensively. She has a mild to moderate increase in bruisability and menorrhagia. Her laboratory tests revealed moderate abnormalities in platelet aggregation, clot retraction, and bleeding time. I have studied several other families with mild hemorrhagic problems in which the only abnormalities were slight prolongation of the bleeding time and minor defects in quantitative clot retraction. They may represent patients with similar but less significant membrane abnormalities. One such family had an autosomal dominant pattern of inheritance.

Local measures and the administration of corticosteroids may be beneficial in controlling minor bleeding, but transfusion of normal platelets is the only way to control significant hemorrhage.

Laboratory findings in thrombasthenia include:

1. Normal platelet count and morphology, with the absence of clumping on peripheral smears made from nonanticoagulated blood.
2. Prolonged bleeding time (slight in heterozygotes).
3. Normal reaction to the tourniquet test.
4. Abnormal quantitative clot retraction (minor abnormality in heterozygotes and mild variant cases).
5. Normal prothrombin consumption test.

6. Absent primary platelet aggregation with ADP, adrenalin, and collagen. Decreased aggregation with ristocetin (mild abnormalities in heterozygotes).
7. Decreased retention in glass bead columns (normal in heterozygotes).
8. Decreased PF_3 availability (normal in heterozygotes).
9. Normal prothrombin time and activated partial thromboplastin time.

Disorders of secondary aggregation or platelet secretion are those in which platelets respond initially to aggregating agents, but subsequent responses associated with the release reaction are impaired. These disorders are not uncommon and result from a variety of abnormalities in the platelet secretory process. They may be inherited or acquired, the latter being more common and usually associated with drug ingestion.

Inherited aggregation defects include *storage pool disease* (Table 2-2), in which platelets have diminished numbers of granules and decreased amounts of granule-bound substances; and *"aspirin-like"* defects (Table 2-2), in which the content of granules is normal but the defect is in the secretory process. Defects of secondary aggregation sometimes occur in association with other congenital abnormalities (e.g., Hermansky-Pudlak, Chediak-Higashi, TAR, Ehlers-Danlos, Wiskott-Aldrich, and May-Hegglin syndromes). The clinical symptoms are generally those of a moderate bleeding disorder, including easy bruisability, excessive bleeding after tooth extractions, menorrhagia, epistaxis, and postpartum bleeding.

Acquired defects of secondary aggregation are usually due to the ingestion of drugs such as aspirin that affect prostaglandin endoperoxide synthesis and thus the release reaction. Since the effect of aspirin is to irreversibly acetylate about 90% of the platelet cyclo-oxygenase, the secretory function of the affected platelet remains impaired throughout its life span (8 to 10 days).

Since platelet aggregation testing is widely available, it is not difficult to identify patients who have abnormalities of aggregation. Hypoaggregability has been more extensively studied than hyperaggregability. Ascertaining the causes of such abnormalities is more difficult. Certainly, in symptomatic patients with acquired disorders, the most important therapeutic step is to identify and remove the cause of the dysfunction when possible. Platelet transfusions can be used when acute hemorrhage is a problem. Since corticosteroids may inhibit platelet aggregation, they are not likely to be helpful in patients with hypoaggregability.

Laboratory findings of diagnostic importance are the following:

1. Normal platelet count and morphology.
2. Normal or prolonged bleeding time (may be more prolonged if patient has an inherited defect and takes aspirin).
3. Normal reaction to the tourniquet test.
4. Normal quantitative clot retraction.
5. Normal prothrombin consumption test.
6. Diminished platelet aggregation with ADP, epinephrine (Adrenalin, Parke-Davis) and collagen, with absence of the second phase. Reduction in maximum aggregation with ristocetin. (Tests may need to be repeated if it is suspected that the patient has ingested drugs.)
7. Spontaneous platelet aggregation in hypercoagulable states; also hyperreactivity to low concentration of aggregating agents.

8. Variable abnormality in retention in glass bead columns (normal in patients whose only problem is aspirin ingestion).
9. Variable abnormality in PF_3 availability.
10. Normal prothrombin time and activated partial thromboplastin time.

Drug Effects on Platelet Function

Drugs affect platelets in many different ways. Table 2-3 gives a list of drugs that cause platelet dysfunction. The best characterized are the effects of drugs that have been used therapeutically as antithrombotic agents. Aspirin and many other nonsteroidal anti-inflammatory agents specifically inhibit the platelet release reaction, but the clinical effectiveness of this inhibition is not well defined. Dipyridamole is known to inhibit platelet phosphodiesterase and may affect in vivo platelet adhesiveness and PF_3 availability, but it has no demonstrable effect on the release reaction. In our laboratory we studied platelet-function tests in normal young adults before and after the ingestion of aspirin, dipyridamole, and ibuprofen (Motrin). Aspirin and Motrin affected only the bleeding times and platelet aggregation. Dipyridamole affected only PF_3 availability. Unless patients have some additional abnormality these drugs do not cause significant bleeding problems.

TABLE 2-3. Drugs Associated with Platelet Dysfunction

Anti-inflammatory agents
  Aspirin
  Other nonsteroidal anti-inflammatory agents
  Corticosteroids
Phosphodiesterase inhibitors
  Methylxanthines (theophylline, caffeine, aminophylline, papaverine)
  Dipyridamole
Antibiotics and antiparasitic agents
  Carbenicillin and related antibiotics
  Nitrofurantoin
  Hydroxychloroquine, chloroquine
Tranquilizers and antipsychotic agents
  Phenothiazines
  Tricyclic antidepressants
Sympathetic blocking agents
  α Blockers
  β Blockers
Miscellaneous agents
  Ethanol, heparin, furosemide, antihistamines, clofibrate, methysergide, reserpine, dextran

Malpass TW, and Harker LA: Acquired disorders of platelet function. Semin Hematol *17*:245, 1980.

Combined Defects of Platelet Function

Combined defects occur most often in patients with inherited disorders who also receive drugs that affect platelet function or in patients with systemic diseases. It is impossible to accurately interpret platelet function tests without an accurate drug and health history. Complex functional platelet defects occur in leukemia, myeloproliferative syndromes, autoimmune disorders, and uremia. Disorders of platelet interaction may occur in DIC, fibrinolytic therapy, and liver disease (due to the presence of fibrinogen-fibrin breakdown products), in paraproteinemias, and with the administration of dextran. Carbenicillin, ampicillin, and cephalothin also affect platelet function by inhibition of the binding of ADP, epinephrine (Adrenalin, Parke-Davis) and other agonists to platelet surfaces.

References

Bachman F: Diagnostic approach to mild bleeding disorders. Semin Hematol *17*:292, 1980.
Lusher JM, and Barnhart MI: Congenital disorders affecting platelets. Semin Thromb Hemostas *4*:123, 1977.
Mueller-Eckhardt C: Idiopathic thrombocytopenic purpura (ITP): clinical and immunological considerations. Semin Thromb Hemostas *3*:125, 1977.
Triplett DA, et al: Platelet Function: Laboratory Evaluation and Clinical Application. Chicago: ASCP, 1978.
Walsh RT: The platelet in von Willebrand's disease: interactions with ristocetin and factor VIII. Semin Thromb Hemostas *2*:105, 1975.
Wantier JL, and Caen JP: Pharmacology of platelet suppressive agents. Semin Thromb Hemostas *5*:293, 1979.
Weiss HJ: Congenital disorders of platelet function. Semin Hematol *17*:228, 1980.

COAGULATION ABNORMALITIES

An abnormality of each of the clotting factors corresponds to a special type of hereditary bleeding syndrome, and in the majority of such disorders, only one clotting factor is reduced or abnormal. The availability of factor-deficient substrates, however, has made it possible to be more accurate in the detection of coagulopathies, and many patients have now been reported who have hereditary multiple factor-deficiencies. In acquired coagulopathies and in the presence of circulating coagulation inhibitors, several factors may appear to be reduced simultaneously. Table 2-4 gives a general classification of some of these disorders, which should be helpful in understanding the following discussion of the individual syndromes.

Of the hereditary coagulopathies, the deficiencies of factors VIII and IX are of sex-linked inheritance, von Willebrand's disease and some dysfibrinogenemias are transmitted as autosomal dominants, and the remainder are autosomal recessive traits.

Inherited Abnormalities of Factors VIII and IX (Hemophilia)

Patients with abnormalities of factors VIII and IX make up the largest number of those having lifelong bleeding disorders. The abnormality of factor VIII, sometimes referred to as hemophilia A, occurs in 1 per 10,000 males and is about 10 times as common as the abnormality of factor IX, hemophilia B. The two deficiencies are indistinguishable clinically, and therefore will be discussed together. Both are inherited disorders, the genes being sex-linked, recessive, and carried on the X chromosome; thus the disease occurs almost exclusively in males. A marriage between an affected male and a normal female can produce only carrier females and normal males. A marriage between a carrier female and a normal male produces both normal and affected males, and both normal and carrier females. Manifestations of both defects range from severe to mild. Among the affected males of a given family, clinical symptoms tend to be fairly uniform. About one third of the subjects have no definite family history, although laboratory testing may identify mothers in such families as carriers. Most often, they result from a long line of transmission of the

TABLE 2-4. Deficiency of Clotting Factors in Hereditary and Acquired Coagulopathies

Clotting Factors	Coagulopathies	
	Hereditary	Acquired
Factor I: Fibrinogen	Afibrinogenemia	Severe liver disease Intravascular clotting Fibrinolysis
Factor II: Prothrombin	Prothrombin deficiency	Liver disease Vitamin K deficiency Anticoagulation Newborn
Factor III: Tissue Thromboplastin		
Factor IV: Calcium		
Factor V: Proaccelerin	Parahemophilia	Severe liver disease Intravascular clotting Fibrinolysis
Factor VII: Proconvertin SPCA	Factor VII deficiency	Liver disease Vitamin K deficiency Anticoagulation Newborn
Factor VIII: Antihemophilic globulin (AHG)	Hemophilia A	Intravascular clotting Fibrinolysis
Factor IX: Christmas factor, PTC	Hemophilia B	Liver disease Vitamin K deficiency
Factor X: Stuart-Prower	Stuart factor deficiency	Anticoagulation Newborn
Factor XI: PTA, Rosenthal factor	PTA deficiency	
Factor XII: Hageman factor	Hageman factor deficiency	
Factor XIII: Fibrin stabilizing factor (FSF)	FSF deficiency	Liver disease Fibrinolysis

Koller F: Clinical and genetic aspects of coagulopathies. Ann Intern Med 62:744, 1965.

hemophilia gene through asymptomatic females without the occurrence of affected males; but new mutations may occur in rare instances. Affected individuals appear to have either normal levels of an inactive protein or reduced levels of a normal one. It is the lack of normal clotting activity that produces the symptoms.

Normal hemostasis following severe trauma requires more than 30% activity levels of either factor VIII or IX (normal range, 50% to 200%). Patients with severe disease have levels below 1% and show repeated spontaneous bleeding and abnormally prolonged bleeding following trauma. Large hematomas and hemarthroses are the most common lesions. Bleeding from the mouth and nose occurs often in children; it is usually associated with minor trauma. Spontaneous hematuria is also common. Tooth extraction and surgical operations are followed by prolonged and severe hemorrhage. In patients with mild defects (levels 6 to 30%), there may be no spontaneous hemorrhage, but excessive bleeding due to tooth extraction commonly occurs. Tonsillectomy is especially to be feared in this group of patients.

In the severely affected patient, all tests of the intrinsic pathway activity are abnormal. The problem is usually that of determining whether factor VIII or factor IX is the deficient factor. The distinction can be made by substitution tests with adsorbed plasma as a source of factor VIII and aged serum as a source of factor IX or by assaying for those factors.

In patients with milder symptoms, the clotting time is usually normal. The reaction to the standard thromboplastin generation test is abnormal when factor levels fall below 20%. The partial thromboplastin time tests show great variability. The activated modification (APTT) is the most sensitive, and the results show variable abnormality with factor levels up to 30%. Unfortunately, the degree of abnormality detected is sometimes so slight that its significance is doubtful. Also, some patients with moderately reduced levels of factor VIII have marked increases in other procoagulants, which compensate for the insufficient amounts of factor VIII and result in normal values in the APTT. In such cases, the thromboplastin generation test or a specific factor assay is much more likely to reflect the true level of the factor.

If a patient has a bleeding history and the only abnormal finding is a slightly prolonged activated partial thromboplastin time, assay procedures for factors VIII and IX should be carried out. With the increased availability of factor VIII and prothrombin complex concentrates, it is essential that these two types of hemophilia be accurately differentiated before instigation of specific blood component therapy.

It is also important to differentiate patients with hemophilia A from those with von Willebrand's disease, many of whom have decreased levels of factor VIII clotting activity, because von Willebrand's patients respond better to cryoprecipitate than to more purified factor VIII concentrates.

Recent experimental work regarding the structure of the factor VIII molecule has resulted in information that is helpful in detecting patients with true hemophilia A and carriers of this defect. In both, the ratio of the level of factor VIII coagulant activity (VIII:C) to the level of factor VIII related antigen (VIII R:Ag) is usually less than 1.0 (approximately 0.5 in carriers and approximately 0.1 in hemophiliacs). In some laboratories, the use of a human antibody to factor VIII:C has allowed the measurement of factor VIII C:Ag. Levels of VIII:C and VIII C:Ag agree well, and in a majority of severe hemophiliacs, both are undetectable. The ratio of factor VIII C:Ag to VIII R:Ag may give better discrimination in the diagnosis of hemophiliac carriers. In hemophilia B (factor IX deficiency), the carrier state is often associated with reduced levels of factor IX coagulant activity.

In patients who have hemophilia A (factor VIII:C deficiency), the ready availability of cryoprecipitate and factor VIII concentrate preparations has revolutionized the therapy. Many children and active adults are on prophylactic doses administered regularly at home. Other patients receive standard doses at the first suggestion that a bleeding episode is starting. It is also possible to maintain adequate levels of factor VIII for dental extraction, surgery, and after trauma, when this is required. The success of such treatment is reflected in a marked reduction in the unemployment rate for adult hemophiliac patients. When dosages are properly selected to attain adequate therapeutic levels, results are excellent except in those hemophiliacs who have inhibitors. The accurate measurement of factor levels is important in the management of such therapy. Prothrombin complex concentrates for patients with hemophilia B (factor IX deficiency) are also readily available and are used in much the same way. Initially such products were considered to be dangerous because they contained activated coagulation enzymes which could produce thrombotic phenomena, but newer products are less active. Specific activated products such as Autoplex and FEIBA may be useful in the treatment of hemophilia A patients who have high titers of inhibitors because the coagulant activity can bypass the reaction that requires factor VIII. Both kinds of concentrates can transmit hepatitis, but the incidence is higher with the use of the prothrombin complex concentrates because of the way in which they are manufactured.

Characteristic laboratory findings in hemophilia include:

1. Normal platelet numbers and morphology and normal platelet function tests.
2. Normal bleeding time (may be significantly prolonged by aspirin).
3. Normal or prolonged clotting time.
4. Usually, increased activated partial thromboplastin time.
5. Usually, abnormal thromboplastin generation test.
   a. Abnormal adsorbed plasma reagent in factor VIII deficiency.
   b. Abnormal serum reagent in factor IX deficiency.
6. Normal or abnormal prothrombin consumption test.
7. Factor VIII and IX clotting-activity assays are diagnostic.
8. Normal factor VIII antigen (VIII R : Ag) by immunoassay.
9. Normal prothrombin time.

Inherited Deficiencies of the Contact Factors

Factor XII (Hageman factor) deficiency had been reported in 81 patients by 1965, and with a few minor exceptions, these persons were found to be remarkably free of hemorrhagic symptoms. The deficiency in most families is inherited as an autosomal recessive characteristic. Persons with factor XII deficiency are primarily a laboratory curiosity and do not demonstrate a bleeding tendency. Recently it was reported that factor XII was present at lower levels in a small group of oriental subjects who were studied (mean, 46%). At least 6 patients with the disorder, including Mr. Hageman in whom it was first recognized, have suffered from myocardial infarctions or thromboembolism.

Factor XI deficiency was first described by Rosenthal et al in 1953, and by 1965 about 200 cases had been reported in the literature. Most of these were in patients of Jewish ancestry, and their symptoms were milder than those of patients with factor VIII or IX deficiency. Transmission is as an incompletely recessive autosomal trait, manifested either as a major defect in homozygotes, with factor XI levels below 20%, or as a minor defect in heterozygotes, with levels from 50 to 65%.

Characteristic laboratory findings for factor XII and factor XI deficiencies include:

1. Normal platelet numbers and morphology and normal platelet function tests.
2. Normal bleeding time.

3. Clotting time more significantly prolonged with factor XII than with factor XI deficiency.
4. Prolonged activated partial thromboplastin time, at least partially corrected by both normal adsorbed plasma and serum reagents but not corrected by prolonged incubation. Correction with normal plasma may not be complete.
5. Abnormal thromboplastin generation test when all reagents are from the patient.
6. Abnormal prothrombin consumption test.
7. Normal prothrombin time.
8. Factor XII and factor XI assays are diagnostic.

Prekallikrein (Fletcher factor) deficiency was first described in 1965 as an inherited abnormality of plasma, which resulted in a prolonged partial thromboplastin time, which could be corrected by prolonged exposure to a surface activating agent. The members of the Fletcher family were asymptomatic and the disorder was of autosomal recessive inheritance. Individuals with moderately prolonged APTT tests in which the abnormality is corrected by prolonged incubation probably have heterozygous prekallikrein deficiencies. A group of such patients were found to have a mean assay result of 54%. Low prekallikrein activity may occur in the newborn and in patients with severe liver disease and uremia.

High molecular weight kininogen (HMWK, Fitzgerald factor, Flaujeac factor) deficiency was described in 1975. The disorder is inherited as an autosomal recessive trait, and patients are totally asymptomatic. Five described kindreds have shown considerable heterogeneity with levels ranging from 0 to 50%.

Laboratory differential diagnosis of prekallikrein and HMWK deficiencies include:
1. Normal platelet numbers and morphology and normal platelet function tests.
2. Normal bleeding time.
3. Prolonged clotting time.
4. In prekallikrein deficiency, the APTT can be corrected by prolonged incubation (10 to 20 minutes) and the test is normal if ellagic acid is the activator. In HMWK deficiency, the APTT is not corrected with prolonged incubation and is abnormal with all types of activators.
5. Normal prothrombin time.
6. Prekallikrein and high molecular weight kininogen assays are diagnostic. There may be a combined deficiency of these factors.

Inherited Abnormalities of Fibrinogen

Afibrinogenemia is a rare, inherited disorder manifested by an almost total lack of circulating fibrinogen. More than 120 cases have been reported. The disorder appears to be inherited as an autosomal recessive, and heterozygous carriers have lower than normal levels of fibrinogen. Consanguinity has been present in over half of the families described. In homozygotes, the blood is completely incoagulable, even on the addition of thrombin. In spite of this, the condition seems to produce milder symptoms than those seen in hemophilia. This is probably due to the fact that the coagulation process proceeds quite normally up to the point of fibrin formation, with the production of adequate amounts of thrombin and the expected changes in the platelets. Afibrinogenemia can be easily distinguished from other deficiency states by the addition of tissue thromboplastin or thrombin to blood or plasma. Blood that does not contain fibrinogen will not clot with either reagent. Blood, plasma, or fibrinogen concentrates may be required during periods of active bleeding or in preparation for surgery. Hemostasis usually may be achieved with fibrinogen levels of 60 to 80 mg/100 ml. At least two patients with this disorder have developed antifibrinogen antibodies following repeated infusions of fibrinogen, and some have shown mild to severe reactions.

Characteristic findings include:

1. Variable mild decrease in platelet numbers.
2. Abnormal platelet aggregation and retention in glass bead columns.
3. Normal or prolonged bleeding time.
4. No clot formation in the clotting time test.
5. No clot formation in the activated partial thromboplastin time test.
6. Normal thromboplastin generation test.
7. No clot formation in the prothrombin time test.
8. No clot formation in the thrombin time test.
9. Assay of fibrinogen reveals its absence. (Traces may be found by immunologic methods.)

Hypofibrinogenemia has been reported in a few patients with mild constitutional bleeding disorders, although the grounds for the recognition of this condition as a true clinical entity are not well established. It is possible that such patients represent examples of dysfibrinogenemia (described below) or the heterozygous state of afibrinogenemia. This condition might be suspected in a patient who has a history of a mild bleeding tendency (usually related to dental extractions) with all coagulation studies normal except for the clot retraction, which shows a moderate increase in red cell fallout. Four patients in one family had levels of fibrinogen that ranged from 120 to 170 mg/dl. In another family, including two generations, 5 of 6 had fibrinogen levels between 60 and 83 mg/dl. Hasselback et al described 5 members of one family in whom the fibrinogen levels varied from 58 to 158 mg/dl. Hampton et al described 2 brothers who had increased capillary fragility, low-normal levels of fibrinogen (137 and 165 mg/dl), and clots with increased solubility in 5 M urea solution (factor XIII deficiency). Routine hemostatic tests in hypofibrinogenemic patients reveal no abnormalities except for the clot retraction, in which there is increased red cell fallout; fibrinogen levels that are slightly to moderately decreased; and qualitative tests for fibrin stabilizing factor, which may show abnormality.

Dysfibrinogenemia is a disorder manifested by the presence in plasma of qualitatively abnormal, functionally defective fibrinogen molecules. More than 55 different functionally defective molecules have now been described and named for the cities in which they were described (e.g., fibrinogen Cleveland, fibrinogen Detroit, fibrinogen Baltimore). The mode of inheritance in these patients seems to be of the incompletely dominant autosomal type and both sexes are equally affected. The fact that most patients appear to have some normal fibrinogen molecules in addition to the abnormal ones suggests that they are heterozygotes. Homozygotes have only abnormal molecules. Affected individuals may be asymptomatic, although some have mild bleeding tendencies. Recurrent thromboembolism has been noted in several kindreds.

Laboratory test results in dysfibrinogenemia include:

1. Normal platelet numbers and morphology.
2. Normal or prolonged bleeding time.
3. Normal or prolonged clotting time (usually normal).
4. Normal or prolonged activated partial thromboplastin time (usually normal).
5. Normal thromboplastin generation test.
6. Prolonged prothrombin time and Stypven time.
7. Markedly prolonged thrombin time, especially when thrombin without calcium is used. Usually not corrected by the addition of normal plasma.
8. Abnormal clot retraction, with a soft friable clot and increased red cell fallout.
9. Clots insoluble in 5 M urea.
10. Normal assay of fibrinogen when quantitative immunologic or physical precipitation methods are used, but decreased levels by methods utilizing the thrombin time.

Inherited Deficiencies of Factors II, V, VII, and X

Factor II (prothrombin) deficiency is among the rarest of the coagulation disorders. It may be caused by decreased production of factor II or by an abnormal molecular structure, and is inherited as an autosomal recessive trait. Less than a dozen cases have been documented, leading to the conclusion that diagnosis of this deficiency should be made with caution. Some cases of dysprothrombinemia have been designated by various proper names (e.g., prothrombin Cardeza). Clinical summaries indicate that hemarthroses are rare, but that epistaxis and bleeding after dental extraction and surgery may be a problem. Levels of factor II vary, but have been found to be as low as 3% and to produce variable prolongation of the prothrombin time from 14 to 73 seconds. It appears that levels of over 40% are required for control of postoperative bleeding, and for this reason, factor concentrates should be much more effective in therapy than is plasma. Unfortunately, the commercially available concentrates containing factors II, VII, IX, and X carry a high risk of causing serum hepatitis.

Characteristic findings are:

1. Normal platelet numbers and morphology and normal platelet function tests.
2. Normal bleeding time.
3. Normal or prolonged clotting time.
4. Normal or prolonged activated partial thromboplastin time.
5. Normal thromboplastin generation test (occasionally abnormal).
6. Variably prolonged prothrombin time (may be nearly normal).
7. Decreased factor II as measured by one-stage or two-stage assay.
8. Normal thrombin time.

Factor V deficiency is also known as parahemophilia and is a rare condition that is transmitted as a highly penetrant and recessive autosomal characteristic. It affects both sexes equally, probably no more frequently than one per 500,000 of the population. In the homozygote the level of factor V is usually below 10%, but heterozygotes have levels of from 22 to 60% and may have 2- to 3-second prolongations of their prothrombin times. Bleeding after trauma, epistaxes, and menorrhagia are the most common symptoms, but some patients have very mild manifestations. Since bleeding can be corrected by a 5 to 10% concentration of factor V, replacement therapy with fresh or fresh frozen plasma is quite satisfactory. Factor concentrates are not available. Test results include:

1. Normal platelet numbers and morphology and normal platelet function tests.
2. Normal or prolonged bleeding time.
3. Normal or prolonged clotting time.
4. Increased activated partial thromboplastin time.
5. Abnormal thromboplastin generation test with patient's adsorbed plasma.
6. Increased prothrombin time, which is corrected by normal adsorbed plasma reagent.
7. Factor V assay is diagnostic.

Factor VII deficiency has been reliably described in about 70 cases. The incidence is believed to be about 1 out of 500,000 persons. The disease appears to be transmitted as a highly penetrant recessive autosomal trait, which produces severe deficiency in the homozygote and moderate deficiency, usually without symptoms, in the heterozygote. Both qualitative and quantitative forms of the deficiency exist. Hemarthrosis, excessive bruising, epistaxis, and menorrhagia may all occur, but the bleeding manifestations are usually mild. Surgical procedures seem to be surprisingly well tolerated. Treatment is complicated by the fact that the circulating half-life of the factor VII is short, being 4 to 6 hours. Characteristic findings include:

1. Normal platelet numbers and morphology and normal platelet function tests.
2. Normal or prolonged bleeding time.
3. Normal clotting time.
4. Normal activated partial thromboplastin time.
5. Normal prothrombin consumption test.
6. Normal thromboplastin generation test.
7. Prolonged prothrombin time that is corrected by normal serum reagent.
8. Normal Stypven time.
9. Factor VII assay is diagnostic.

Factor X deficiency occurs in a heterogeneous group of patients. Some apparently completely lack the factor; whereas others have either a normal or a decreased amount of a factor that reacts immunologically with factor X antibody, but is functionally inactive. The rate of incidence and bleeding history are similar to those of factor VII deficiency; and it is likewise transmitted as a highly penetrant, recessive autosomal characteristic. Clinical manifestations are generally mild although there is some evidence that a blood level in excess of 10% is required for hemostatic efficiency. The symptomatic patient should have adequate replacement therapy with plasma or a factor concentrate. This is facilitated by the fact that factor X has a long half-life (about 25 to 60 hours). Pregnancy and anovulatory drugs have been known to produce spontaneous remissions of bleeding problems in persons with this defect. It has been suggested that some patients with slight consistent prolongation of their prothrombin time tests (i.e., 16 seconds) may be heterozygous for factor X deficiency. Characteristic finding are the following:

1. Normal platelet numbers and morphology and normal platelet function tests.
2. Normal bleeding time (rarely prolonged).
3. Normal or prolonged clotting time.
4. Prolonged activated partial thromboplastin time corrected by normal serum reagent.
5. Abnormal thromboplastin generation test with patient's serum reagent.
6. Prolonged prothrombin time corrected by normal serum reagent.
7. Normal or prolonged Stypven time.
8. Factor X assay is diagnostic.

Factor XIII Deficiency

Even though factor XIII was discovered in 1944 by Robbins, a patient with a hereditary deficiency of the factor was not described until 1960 (Duckert et al). Since then, at least 10 more cases have been reported and they were all characterized by umbilical bleeding, hematomata, ecchymoses, bleeding after cuts, and defective wound healing. The defect appears to be inherited as an autosomal recessive, but sex-linked inheritance has also been reported. Homozygotes have levels of factor XIII that are near zero, and in some cases, reduced levels have been shown in parents. The hemostatically effective level is about 5%, and in patients given prophylactic transfusion a level of 0.5% appears to be sufficient. Acquired defects of factor XIII activity have been described in some patients with liver disease, metastatic carcinoma, leukemia, pernicious anemia, myeloma, agammaglobulinemia, lead poisoning, and collagen diseases.

For diagnostic purposes, thromboelastography is certainly the best method for detecting a lack or reduction of the factor. There is a direct and quantitative relationship between the amplitude of the thromboelastogram and the content of factor XIII, a diminution to 60% or less being detectable in the test system. Since thromboelastography is not available in many laboratories, however, a second choice is the qualitative test for fibrin stabilizing factor (clot stability in 5 M urea). This test is not nearly as sensitive as the thromboelastogram, since it takes only about 1 to 2% of factor XIII to produce a clot that is insoluble in the urea solution. All tests except the thromboelastogram and qualitative and quantitative tests for fibrin stabilizing factor are normal in most patients; however, in one family, the fibrinogen levels were low and capillary fragility was increased.

Other Rare Hereditary Coagulation Disorders

Passavoy factor deficiency is a mild inherited hemorrhagic disorder which is the result of a specific abnormality in the intrinsic pathway. It is manifested by a slightly prolonged activated partial thromboplastin time and normal levels of all known coagulation factors.

Deficiencies of α-2-antiplasmin and α-1-antitrypsin have also been described. Both were associated with lifelong bleeding disorders. Deficiency of antithrombin III is associated with thromboembolic problems.

Inherited Multiple-Coagulation-Factor Deficiencies

The first comprehensive review of inherited multiple-coagulation-factor deficiencies was published in 1981 (Soff and Leven). Two types of multiple-factor deficiencies were described. The first type is due to the coincidental concurrence of more than one disorder and occurs very rarely. The second type is due to a single heritable disorder associated with deficiencies of two or more factors. The most commonly reported multiple-factor deficiency is combined factor V and factor VIII deficiency, which in most instances, is an example of the second type since it appears to be due to a deficiency of an inhibitor of protein C (protein C is known to inactivate factors V and VIII). Other familial multiple-factor deficiencies are listed in Table 2-5. There are important practical reasons for considering these syndromes when doing hemostasis work-ups. Often, laboratory investigation is terminated when a deficiency of a single coagulation factor is detected. Appropriate therapy depends on the identification of all deficient factors, since replacement therapy now often involves the use of isolated factor concentrates.

TABLE 2-5. Familial Multiple Factor Deficiencies

	Deficient Factors	Pathogenesis
FMFD I	V, VIII	Protein C Inhibitor deficiency
FMFD II	VII, IX	Unknown
FMFD III	II, VII, IX, X	Deficient Γcarboxylation of glutamic acid
FMFD IV	VII, VIII	Unknown
FMFD V	VII, IX, XI	Unknown
FMFD VI	IX, XI	Unknown

Acquired Combined Deficiencies of the Vitamin K-Dependent Factors

Vitamin K-dependent factors (II, VII, IX, and X) are synthesized in the liver and share the property that synthesis of their active forms requires vitamin K. When this vitamin is deficient, abnormal, hypofunctional analogues of these factors are synthesized, which lack normal clotting activity. Activity levels of all these factors are depressed in the neonatal period (hemorrhagic disease of the newborn); by treatment with coumarin-type oral anticoagulants; in severe liver failure; and in conditions that result in impaired dietary intake or absorption of vitamin K (malabsorption syndromes, obstructive jaundice, prolonged antibiotic therapy, and total parenteral nutrition). In these acquired deficiencies, activity of all four factors tends to be diminished simultaneously, although not necessarily to the same extent.

All newborn infants have deficiencies of factors II, VII, IX, and X, and the concentrations of these factors fall even lower during the first few days of life, reaching their lowest levels by about the third day. Such deficiencies are more marked in premature infants and in those born to mothers who have been on inadequate diets during pregnancy. In a small percentage, there will be significant hemorrhagic manifestations on the second or third day of life, the most common symptoms being persistent bleeding from the umbilical stump, epistaxis, and gastrointestinal hemorrhage. If bleeding is severe, transfusion with fresh whole blood may be required, but usually, the administration of small doses of vitamin K will correct the coagulation defect within a few hours.

A much more common cause of an acquired deficiency of the vitamin K-dependent factors is the use of coumarin-type anticoagulant drugs. When such drugs are ingested, changes may not be detected in blood coagulation for a day or two. Because of the differences in the half-lives of these factors, their activity levels begin to fall at different times and rates. A decrease in factor VII is noted first, followed by decreases in factors IX and X, and finally II. The degree of depression is dependent primarily on drug dosage, the levels gradually returning to normal when the coumarin-type drug is discontinued. The administration of vitamin K_1 shortens the recovery period. Patients have been known to take oral anticoagulants secretly in order to produce hemorrhagic symptoms that will require the attention and care of a physician. We have seen several such cases, particularly among nurses and hospital personnel to whom such medications are available.

Liver disease, besides producing deficiencies of the vitamin-K dependent factors, may also cause depression of factor V, abnormalities in fibrinogen, thrombocytopenia, and chronic fibrinolysis. The parenteral administration of vitamin K_1 is usually not helpful unless the problem is one of obstructive jaundice with impaired absorption of vitamin K.

Expected laboratory findings in this group of deficiencies include:
1. Normal platelet numbers and morphology (except in liver disease, when thrombocytopenia may occur). Platelet function tests are usually normal.
2. Normal bleeding time.
3. Normal clotting time.
4. Prolonged partial thromboplastin time in marked deficiencies.
5. Abnormal prothrombin time, at least partially correctable with normal serum reagent.
6. Assays for factors II, VII, IX, and X are diagnostic.

Acquired Inhibitors of Blood Coagulation

Acquired inhibitors of blood coagulation, also known as circulating anticoagulants, are pathologic substances in blood that directly inhibit clotting factors or their reactions and are endogenously produced. Well-documented inhibitors include the following:
1. Factor VIII : C inhibitors in
    a. Hemophilia A.
    b. Patients with immunologic problems.
    c. Women after childbirth.
    d. Miscellaneous older patients.

2. Factor VIII R : WF inhibitors (rare).
3. Factor IX inhibitors in hemophilia B and, rarely, in previously normal persons.
4. Factor V inhibitors in factor V deficiency and in previously normal persons (rare).
5. Factor VII, XI, and XII inhibitors (very rare).
6. Factor I inhibitors in patients with afibrinogenemia.
7. Factor XIII inhibitors in patients with factor XIII deficiency and in previously normal persons (rare).
8. Inhibitors of the thrombin-fibrinogen reaction (FDP and paraproteins).
9. The "lupus" inhibitor.

Most factor VIII inhibitors are immunoglobulins of the IgG type that inactivate factor VIII by means of a time-and-temperature-dependent reaction and are specific for the portion of the factor VIII molecule that provides the clotting activity (VIII:C). From 5 to 20% of all patients with hemophilia A who receive replacement therapy eventually develop such inhibitors, usually before the age of 10 years. This occurs in severe hemophiliacs who are cross-reacting material (CRM)-negative (without any material in their plasmas capable of neutralizing human factor VIII inhibitors). Simple mixing techniques may miss inhibitors of low titer, so detection and quantitation are best accomplished by measuring specifically the level of factor VIII activity after incubating test plasma with a standard plasma of known factor VIII level. The inhibitor activity is reported in standardized units ("Bethesda" units). The type of bleeding in hemophiliac patients who develop the inhibitor is usually not altered, but bleeding may be found to be more protracted and less responsive to replacement therapy. Once formed, the antibody levels run a variable course. Reexposure to factor VIII generally produces a rapid rise in inhibitor titer, becoming apparent 2 to 4 days following exposure and reaching a maximum within about 2 weeks. In the absence of rechallenge with factor VIII, inhibitor levels tend to fall slowly. Occasionally, high levels are maintained for long periods, and there are a few instances in which such inhibitors have disappeared entirely.

Replacement therapy with factor VIII may require the administration of large quantities and is only practical in patients with low levels of inhibitor activity. To prevent elevation of the inhibitor titer, one should avoid administration of factor VIII in such patients, whenever possible. In patients with higher levels, it is often necessary to use an activated prothrombin complex concentrate.

The physical and chemical characteristics of factor VIII inhibitors that develop in patients suffering from immunologic states, in women after childbirth, and in otherwise normal persons resemble those of the inhibitors that occur in hemophiliacs. Clinically, such patients develop a hemorrhagic state closely resembling hemophilia but have residual factor VIII:C activity despite the presence of their inhibitors, which are usually of low titer. The inhibitor activity is not increased by administration of factor VIII concentrates, but such therapy is usually ineffective. Prednisone and cytoxan have been used effectively in the treatment of some patients.

Inhibitors of factor VIII R:WF have been detected in patients with von Willebrand's disease and in previously normal persons. Inhibitors of factor IX have been observed in an average of 5% of all patients with factor IX deficiency, and rarely, in previously normal persons. Factor IX inhibitors are of the IgG type, but differ from factor VIII inhibitors in that they act instantaneously.

Immunoglobulin inhibitors of factor V, although not common, have been described frequently enough, particularly in postoperative patients who have received transfusions or streptomycin, that they should always be considered in the differential diagnosis of an obscure bleeding problem. Such inhibitors seldom result in serious hemorrhage and disappear spontaneously in most cases. They have also been reported in patients with hereditary factor V deficiency. Inhibitors of factors VII, XI, and XII have also been described.

Several cases of inhibitor production have occurred in patients with afibrinogenemia following replacement therapy. These inhibitors cause an abnormally rapid disappearance of infused fibrinogen. Factor XIII inhibitors occur rarely in deficient patients and also in patients who have received isoniazid. Fibrinogen-fibrin degradation products (FDP), when formed in excess during intravascular clotting, interfere with the polymerization of fibrin monomers by producing soluble fibrin monomer complexes (SFMC) that clot slowly or not at all. They can usually be neutralized by protamine sulfate, and their presence is probably responsible for inhibitor activity that has been attributed to heparin-like anticoagulants.

Increased amounts of polyclonal immunoglobulins or monoclonal paraproteins, such as occur in multiple myeloma and Waldenström's macroglobulinemia, may inhibit coagulation by interference with polymerization of fibrin monomers. The thrombin time is most significantly affected, but if the anticoagulant effect is great enough, this will be reflected in slight to moderate prolongation of the prothrombin time and in tests of the intrinsic pathway such as the activated partial thromboplastin time. There is, however, no evidence that these proteins interfere during early stages of coagulation. When the effect is due to the large quantity of immunoglobulin molecules, it can frequently be decreased by testing diluted plasma.

Inhibitors of the "lupus" type were originally reported in patients with systemic lupus, but have now been detected in a wide variety of subjects, some of whom have no known physical disorder and no bleeding problem. It has been said that such inhibitors may be the most common cause of prolonged activated partial thromboplastin time tests. They are immunoglobulins of either the IgG or IgM class and act instantaneously. Most evidence suggests that they interact with the phospholipid component of platelets (PF_3) or with tissue thromboplastin (TF) and thus may interfere at the three steps in the coagulation cascade where phospholipid is known to be necessary (IX_a, VIII, Ca^{++}, PF_3, X reaction; X_a, V, Ca^{++}, PF_3, II reaction; and TF, VII_a, X, Ca^{++}, reaction). Even though such inhibitors interact with the phospholipid component of the tissue thromboplastin reagent used in the prothrombin time test, the prothrombin time test is often normal unless the thromboplastin reagent is diluted. This is because the reagent is present in great excess in the test. Patients with very high titers of inhibitor or with a concomitant deficiency of factor II (which has been reported to be deficient in some patients, particularly those with bleeding symptoms) may have prolonged prothrombin times in addition to prolonged APTT's. Since abnormal bleeding rarely occurs, the most important laboratory problem is the proper identification of such inhibitors, particularly when abnormal test results have been found during routine preoperative screening. Corticosteroids and immunosup-

TABLE 2-6.   Comparison of Factor VIII and "Lupus" Inhibitors

Factor VIII Inhibitors	*"Lupus" Inhibitors*
1. Bleeding often severe	1. Bleeding uncommon; thromboembolic manifestations may occur
2. APTT prolonged	2. APTT prolonged
3. PT normal	3. PT may be normal; always prolonged with diluted thromboplastin reagent
4. Thrombin time normal	4. Thrombin time reportedly prolonged in some cases
5. Inhibitory effect in mixtures of test and normal plasma is time-and-temperature dependent	5. Inhibitory effect in mixtures of test and normal plasma is instantaneous and often not marked
6. Factor II normal by specific assay	6. Factor II may be decreased by specific assay
7. One-stage assays for factors XII, XI, IX and VIII give low levels with standard dilutions, but may give higher levels with greater dilutions. In severe hemophilia A, patients' factor VIII levels are very low at all dilutions	7. One-stage assays for factor XII, XI, IX and VIII give low levels with standard dilutions, but may giver higher levels with greater dilutions

pressive drugs have been effective in many symptomatic patients. A comparison of factor VIII and "lupus" type inhibitors is shown in Table 2-6.

The presence of excessive circulating inhibitors should always be considered (1) when patients with a known hemorrhagic diathesis suddenly become refractory to therapy, (2) when a coagulopathy develops in a previously healthy person, and (3) when certain coagulation tests give contradictory results that are not in agreement with the pattern known for a typical coagulation-deficiency disease. Some characteristic findings are the following:

1. Normal platelet numbers and morphology and normal platelet function tests.
2. Prolonged whole blood and plasma clotting times with almost all types of inhibitors.
3. Prolonged activated partial thromboplastin time with almost all types of inhibitors.
4. Variable abnormalities in the thromboplastin generation test.
5. Prolonged prothrombin time with inhibitors of factors V, VII, and I, and with some "lupus" inhibitors.
6. Prolonged thrombin time with all inhibitors related to fibrin formation, except the factor XIII inhibitors.
7. Lack of complete correction of abnormal clotting tests by the addition of normal plasma.
8. Variable abnormalities in specific factor assays. Often multiple factors appear to be decreased when one-stage assays are used.

References

Bachman F: Diagnostic approach to mild bleeding disorders. Semin Hematol *17*:292, 1980.
Borchgrevink CF, et al: A study of a case of congenital hypoprothrombinemia. Br J Haematol *5*:294, 1959.

Conrad FG, Breneman WL, and Grisham DB: A clinical evaluation of plasma thromboplastin antecedent (PTA deficiency). Ann Intern Med 62:885, 1965.

Duckert R, Jung E, and Shmerling DH: A hitherto undescribed congenital hemorrhagic diathesis probably due to fibrin stabilizing factor deficiency. Thromb Diath Haemorrh 5:179, 1960.

Feinstein DI, and Rapaport SI: Acquired inhibitors of blood coagulation. Prog Hemost Thromb 1:72, 1972.

Graham JB: Genotype assignment (carrier detection) in the hemophilias. Clin Haematol 8:115, 1979.

Hampton JW, Bird RM, and Hammarsten DM: Defective fibrinase activity in two brothers. J Lab Clin Med 65:469, 1965.

Hasselback R, Marion RB, and Thomas JW: Congenital hypofibrinogenemia in five members of a family. Can Med Assoc J 88:19, 1963.

Hathaway WE, Belhasen LP, and Hathaway HS: Evidence for a new plasma thromboplastin factor I. Case report, coagulation studies and physicochemical properties. Blood 26:521, 1965.

Hathaway WE, et al: Clinical and physiologic studies of two siblings with prekallikrein (Fletcher factor) deficiency. Am J Med 60:654, 1976.

Hattersley PG, and Hayse D: The effect of increased contact activation time on the activated partial thromboplastin time. Am J Clin Pathol 66:479, 1976.

Herbst KD, Rappaport SI, Kenoyer DG, et al: Syndrome of an acquired inhibitor of factor VIII responsive to cyclophosphamide and prednisone. Ann Intern Med 95:575, 1981.

Houghie C, et al: The Passavoy defect. N Engl J Med 298:1045, 1978.

Kasper CK, Aledort LM, and Counts RB: A more uniform measurement of factor VIII inhibitors. Thromb Diath Haemorrh 34:869, 1975, letter.

Koller F: Clinical and genetic aspects of coagulopathies. Ann Intern Med 62:744, 1965.

Lechner K, Niessner H, and Thaler E: Coagulation abnormalities in liver disease. Semin Thromb Hemostas 4:40, 1977.

Lowe GDO, and Forbes CD: Laboratory diagnosis of congenital coagulation defects. Clin Haematol 8:79, 1979.

Mammen EF: Congenital abnormalities of the fibrinogen molecule. Semin Thromb Hemostas 1:184, 1974.

Margolius A, Jackson DP, and Ratnoff OD: Circulating anticoagulants: A study of 40 cases and a review of the literature. Medicine 40:145, 1961.

Nilsson IM, and Holmberg L: von Willebrand's disease today. Clin Haematol 8:147, 1979.

Nussbaum M, and Morse BS: Plasma fibrin stabilizing factor activity in various diseases. Blood 23:669, 1964.

Owren PA: The coagulation of blood. Investigations of a new clotting factor. Acta Med Scand, Supplement 194, 1947.

Peake IR, et al: Carrier detection in haemophilia A by immunological measurement of factor VIII related antigen (VIII R Ag) and factor VIII clotting antigen (VIII C Ag). Br J Haematol 48:651, 1981.

Penner JA, and Kelly RE: Management of patients with factor VIII or IX inhibitors. Semin Thromb Hemostas 1:386, 1975.

Schleider MA, et al: A clinical study of the lupus anticoagulant. Blood 48:499, 1976.

Shapiro SS, and Hultin M: Acquired inhibitors to the blood coagulation factors. Semin Thromb Hemostas 1:336, 1975.

Shapiro SS: Antibodies to blood coagulation factors. Clin Haematol 8:207, 1979.

Soff GA, and Levin J: Familial multiple coagulation factor deficiencies. Semin Thromb Hemostas 7:112, 1981.

Wintrobe MM, et al: Clinical Hematology, 8th ed. Philadelphia, Lea & Febiger, 1982.

COMPLEX ABNORMALITIES OF HEMOSTASIS AND THROMBOSIS
Hemorrhagic Disorders Associated with Common Systemic Diseases

Bleeding in patients with liver disease may result from multiple coagulation defects, thrombocytopenia, excessive fibrinolysis, or a combination of these abnormalities. Associated gastrointestinal bleeding is more often due to local causes such as acute gastritis, peptic ulcer, or esophageal varices, but such bleeding may be aggravated by the hemostatic defects. Deficiencies of factors II, VII, IX, and X resulting solely from liver damage do not respond to the administration of vitamin K; however, some improvement may occur if interference with vitamin K adsorption has contributed to the deficiency.

Uremia may result in a slight decrease in platelet count and an acquired defect in platelet function. Deficiencies of factors I, V, and VII have been described, plus the presence of a circulating anticoagulant.

Patients with myeloproliferative diseases are prone to operative and postoperative hemorrhage, probably due mainly to impaired platelet function. Factors I and V may also be decreased, and the whole blood clot has a pronounced cohesive instability.

Since platelets and factors V and VIII deteriorate significantly during storage of blood, hemostasis may become impaired when systemic diseases require rapid transfusion of large volumes of bank blood. For this reason, when more than 10 units of blood are required in a 24 hour period, 1 of every 3 units should be fresh blood, or platelet concentrates and fresh-frozen plasma should be supplied in addition. Calcium chloride may also be given to avoid cardiac dysfunction due to hypocalcemia.

Hemostatic Problems Associated with Open Heart Surgery

Many instances of bleeding associated with open heart surgery are clearly due to inadequate surgical technique; however, a significant number are due to alterations in hemostasis associated with extracorporeal circulation and the use of anticoagulant therapy. Both thrombocytopenia and significant defects in platelet function are commonly found in patients who bleed excessively. The most common coagulation-factor defects are those of factors II, V, and VIII. DIC can occur during cardiopulmonary bypass and manipulation of cardiac tissue, and increased fibrinogenolysis has been attributed to pump-induced activation of the plasminogen-plasmin system. Over-medication with heparin, heparin rebound, inadequate protamine neutralization, and protamine excess have rarely been clearly documented as causes of bleeding problems. Predisposing factors to excess bleeding include (1) longer pump runs, (2) prior ingestion of coumarin-type anticoagulants, and (3) cyanotic heart disease.

It is extremely important to determine preoperatively whether a patient has an already existing bleeding diathesis or is taking drugs that may contribute to abnormal hemostasis. Minimal preoperative screening tests should include a platelet count, bleeding time, activated partial thromboplastin time, and thrombin time. If bleeding occurs intra- or postoperatively, it is essential to test for evidence of heparin excess and hyperfibrinolysis. Platelets may be given empirically because of the common occurrence of platelet functional defects.

Hypercoagulability

Hypercoagulability can be defined as an altered state of the circulating blood that requires a smaller quantity of clot-promoting stimuli to induce intravascular coagulation than is required to produce comparable thrombosis in a normal subject. This definition can include any changes in blood components that can be considered pathogenetically important in the development of intravascular thromboses (Table 2-7).

Platelet numbers may be increased in hypercoagulability and thrombocytosis is clinically important in the thrombohemorrhagic problems associated with myeloproliferative syndromes. "Reactive" thrombocytosis does not appear to be pathogenetically important. Increased platelet adhesiveness and aggregability may contribute to the thrombotic potential even when platelet numbers are normal. Such

TABLE 2-7.   Laboratory Changes Reported To Be
Associated With Hypercoagulability

I. Increased platelet numbers or reactivity
$\uparrow$ Circulating platelet aggregates
Spontaneous aggregation
Absence of disaggregation with weak ADP
$\uparrow$ Retention in glass bead columns
$\downarrow$ Response to antiplatelet drugs
Shortened bleeding time

II. Decreased platelet survival

III. Changes in levels of activity of coagulation factors or inhibitors
$\uparrow$ Factors VIII, V, and I (nonspecific)
Change in ratio of immunologic and biologic VIII
Increased rate of thrombin generation
Changes in thrombokinetogram
No direct assays for activated forms of XII, XI, IX, X, II, VII
$\downarrow$ AT III or molecular alteration

IV. Increased fibrinogen turnover (not very sensitive)

V. Appearance of fibrinopeptide A (RIA)

VI. Circulating soluble fibrin monomer complexes (3P, ethanol gel, cryofibrinogen)

VII. Decreased fibrinolysis (with venous occlusion); Increased antiplasmins

VIII. Presence of fibrinogen-fibrin degradation products (nonspecific)

functional abnormalities of platelets have been described in patients with diabetes, hyperlipoproteinemia, and angina pectoris. Platelet survival has been reported to be reduced in a wide variety of patients, particularly those with arterial and valvular disorders. This could be due to alterations in vascular endothelial surfaces as well as in platelets. In thrombotic thrombocytopenic purpura, there appears to be a plasma abnormality that is related to the formation of platelet thrombi. Increased plasma levels of platelet factor 4 and β-thromboglobulin may be found in patients in whom platelets have been activated in vivo.

Increased levels of almost every known coagulation factor have been described at some time in patients with a tendency to thrombosis; however, there is very little concrete evidence that such increased levels alone lead to an increased rate of fibrin formation. The levels of factors V, VIII, and fibrinogen are increased during inflammatory processes because they are acute-phase reactant proteins; but this probably represents a response to such processes rather than the cause of the thrombosis that may accompany them. Levels of several coagulation factors increase during pregnancy and in individuals taking estrogens, but demonstrable direct effects of these increases are lacking, even though the incidence of thrombotic events in both situations is increased.

Decreased levels of antithrombin III (AT III) are known to be associated with an increased tendency to thrombosis. Thrombotic problems have been reported in several families with AT III levels of 40 to 50%. Levels of AT III fall during active thrombotic states, especially in DIC, and this may perpetuate the thrombotic tendency. AT III is also mildly decreased in individuals taking estrogen.

Several methods can be used to detect intravascular fibrin formation through the measurement of products of the fibrinogen-to-fibrin conversion reaction. If such tests are positive, this is not specific evidence of an on-going hypercoagulable state, but rather evidence that an episode of intravascular coagulation has occurred.

Normally, the euglobulin-lysis time of plasma is significantly decreased if a blood sample is drawn after venous occlusion for 5 minutes with a blood pressure cuff. The effect occurs because of the release of activator from the venous endothelium, and if it does not, fibrinolytic activity can be assumed to be diminished. Plasminogen levels may be increased when activator activity is diminished or when antiplasmin is increased, whereas they are usually low immediately following periods of active fibrinolysis.

We have recently selected a group of tests that are most likely to give evidence of the presence of a hypercoagulable state. Any of the following may be helpful.

1. Increased platelet numbers with associated abnormalities in morphology and/or platelet function.
2. Increased platelet retention in glass bead columns (when Adeplat T columns are used).
3. Increased platelet aggregation with low concentrations of collagen.
4. Absence of rapid platelet disaggregation after weak ADP stimulation.
5. Increased levels of PF_4 and/or β-thromboglobulin in plasma.
6. Increased speed of thrombin generation (a decreased thrombin-generation-time test, TGTT).
7. Decreased antithrombin III (AT III).
8. Presence of soluble fibrin monomer complexes (SFMC) in plasma (protamine sulfate, ethanol gelation, or cryofibrinogen tests).
9. Presence of fibrinogen-fibrin degradation products (FDP) in serum.
10. Prolonged euglobulin clot lysis test, especially after venous occlusion.
11. Increased levels of antiplasmin. Plasminogen may be high or low.
12. Increased levels of factors I, V, and VIII (of questionable significance).
13. Resistance to anticoagulant therapy.

In a new research project, we are measuring platelet numbers, platelet retention in Adeplat T columns, aggregation with low concentrations of collagen, the TGTT, and AT III.

Intravascular Coagulation

Normally, blood does not coagulate within the uninjured vascular system. Under a variety of pathologic conditions, however, intravascular clotting can occur. The process may be (1) localized, as in the formation of arterial and venous thrombi, (2) embolic, or (3) generalized in the microcirculation, as in the syndrome of disseminated intravascular coagulation (DIC) (Figure 2-1). Thrombotic processes may develop acutely or slowly and may be of mild or severe degree. The location of localized venous and arterial thrombi and emboli is of central importance in determining the symptoms that will be produced. With DIC, the severity and duration of the process are of major importance, since coagulation usually occurs throughout the microvasculature.

THE SCOPE OF THE PROBLEM

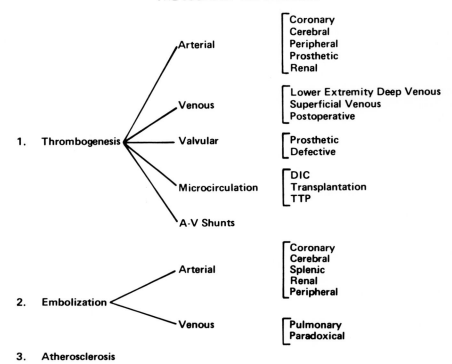

Figure 2-1. Classification of thromboembolic processes.

Many unrelated factors help to prevent pathologic intravascular clotting, such as (1) the "nonwettable" and fibrinolytic surface of the vascular endothelium, (2) the release of prostacyclin (PGI_2) from stimulated endothelial cells, (3) the slow rate of clotting via the intrinsic pathway, (4) the avidity of the reticuloendothelial system for circulating activated coagulant substances, and (5) the availability of naturally occurring plasmatic inhibitors of blood coagulation. Normal flow patterns and lack of stasis are also extremely important; however, in many instances these mechanisms are ineffective and the normal fluidity of blood is lost. Figure 2-2 demonstrates the many factors involved in the development of a tendency to thrombosis.

Localized Intravascular Thrombosis and Thromboembolism

Localized venous thrombi occur most often in veins of the lower extremity, usually in areas of trauma, inflammation, or where blood flow is slowed or obstructed. Stasis occurs regularly with inactivity, and the presence of varicose veins is a common contributing factor. Since increased coagulability is associated with the period of late pregnancy and delivery and also with surgical procedures, there is a significant occurrence of postpartum and postoperative venous thrombosis in the lower extremities at these times. Such processes, if extensive, are often associated with pulmonary embolization.

THE PROBLEM

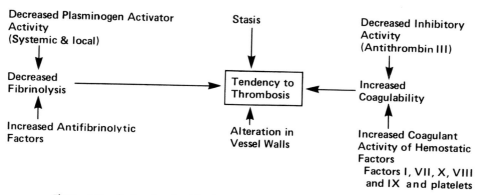

Figure 2-2. Factors involved in the development of a tendency to thrombosis.

Localized arterial thrombi most often occur when there is an accumulation of platelet-fibrin masses at sites of abnormalities that have developed in vessel walls. Common sites are the coronary and cerebral arteries, where thrombosis results in myocardial infarction and strokes. Embolization may occur from thrombotic masses that develop at such sites as the common carotid artery or other cerebral arteries with the occurrence of transient ischemic attacks. Peripheral arterial occlusion may occur due to embolization from thrombotic masses in arterial vessels such as the aorta. Increased coagulability and decreased fibrinolysis may be contributory factors.

Disseminated Intravascular Coagulation (DIC)

The syndrome of disseminated intravascular coagulation differs from the formation of localized thrombi in veins and arteries in that it is generalized and results in the widespread deposition of thrombi in the microcirculation of all organs. DIC is always a response to an underlying process that provokes a generalized activation of the hemostatic mechanism, leading to the evolution of thrombin and deposition of fibrin. Fortunately, this results in a series of protective mechanisms that the body employs to defend itself against the generalized clotting that would occur in the presence of unchecked thrombin.

Stimuli that provoke DIC vary in type, strength, and duration of their action and produce a variety of clinical syndromes (Table 2-8). As shown in Figure 2-3, those stimuli that promote clotting primarily by surface activation due to endothelial damage include infectious agents, heat, anoxemia, acidosis, and dietary lipids. Isolated stimulation of platelets is more likely to be brought about by drugs, antigen-antibody complexes, viruses, and endotoxin. A close interrelationship exists, however, between endothelial damage and platelet stimulation, since platelets tend to adhere to the collagen of damaged vessel walls and aggregate there; also, the intrinsic coagulation pathway is affected both by the activation of factor XII on endothelial and platelet surfaces and by the presence of available platelet factor 3.

A more common event is for tissue thromboplastin to initiate clotting by the more rapid extrinsic pathway; this may occur in the absence of endothelial and platelet

TABLE 2-8.   Etiologic Agents and Related Clinical Syndromes
of Disseminated Intravascular Coagulation

Experimentally Produced	Possible Clinical Syndromes
Thrombin or thromboplastin intravenously	Abruptio placenta Dead fetus syndrome Abortion Trauma Surgery with tissue damage Disseminated malignancy Snake venoms Shock (surgical or infectious)
Hemolyzed blood intravenously	Incompatible blood transfusion Acute hemolytic anemia
Amniotic fluid intravenously	Amniotic fluid embolism
Bacterial endotoxin intravenously	Septicemia Shwartzman reaction
Antigen-antibody complexes	Immune diseases Purpura fulminans
Viremia	Hemorrhagic fevers
Thermal damage to vessels	Heat stroke
Blood stasis and surface activation	Shock Hemangiomas Dissecting aneurysms Cardiopulmonary bypass

damage. Common sources of tissue thromboplastin include hemolyzed RBCs and placental, neoplastic, and traumatized tissue. The initiation of acute DIC by tissue thromboplastin is most likely to occur during rapid intravascular hemolysis and obstetrical and surgical emergencies. A more chronic form is associated with malignancies, since the release of tissue thromboplastin usually occurs slowly from neoplastic tissue. One of the common causes of DIC is gram-negative sepsis, which involves not only coagulation via the intrinsic and extrinsic pathways, but also the release of vasoactive kinins (Figure 2-4).

Fortunately, active local fibrinolysis almost invariably accompanies microvascular clotting, and excess thrombin is inactivated rapidly, so the process can be controlled if the initiating stimulus can be eliminated. DIC may be exaggerated when the reticulothelial system becomes overloaded and when antithrombin III is decreased. When fibrinolytic activity is insufficient to bring about rapid removal of clots, infarction and necrosis of tissue may result. When, however, the drive toward clotting is minimal due to depletion of procoagulant proteins, and exaggerated secondary fibrinolysis occurs, the clinical manifestations are more likely to be those of hemorrhage (Figure 2-5).

Laboratory abnormalities vary, depending on whether the condition is acute or chronic, mild or severe, compensated, decompensated, or over-compensated (Table 2-9). Both the clinical picture and laboratory results may change by the hour as the situation worsens or improves. Tests can be divided into three groups, as in Table 2-10, relative to their specificity and sensitivity. It is important to emphasize that

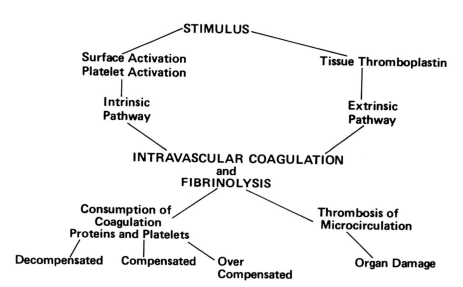

Figure 2-3.   Kinds of stimuli that promote intravascular coagulation and related clinical problems.

serial testing is important to determine both the evolution of the process and the response to therapy. The most useful group of tests includes the following:
1.   Fibrinogen concentration.
2.   Platelet count.
3.   Prothrombin time.
4.   FDP.
5.   Plasma protamine paracoagulation (3P) test.

It is important to mention that all tests that are included in initial testing may not need to be repeated when follow-up testing is done. Tests that are likely to show rapid change are the most useful clinically. These are the prothrombin time and fibrinogen concentration.

Antithrombotic Therapy

The coumarin-type oral anticoagulants interfere with the vitamin K-mediated hepatic synthesis of factors II, VII, IX, and X. The resultant deficiency state is discussed earlier in this chapter as an example of an acquired combined deficiency of the vitamin K-dependent factors. The prothrombin-time test is satisfactory for monitoring the use of these drugs. With a mild to moderate prolongation of the

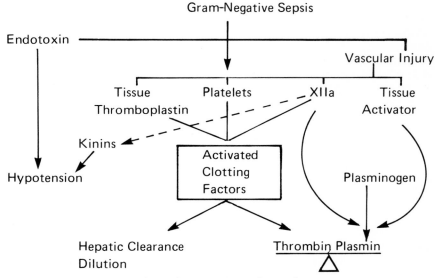

Figure 2-4. Gram-negative sepsis.

prothrombin time, there may be little change in the activated partial thromboplastin time, but more significant alterations produce parallel changes in both tests. Hemorrhage is the most common complication of oral anticoagulant therapy.

Heparin has a different anticoagulant effect: it inhibits coagulation immediately after being administered. A plasma cofactor (antithrombin III) is required for its anticoagulant effect. Heparin molecules attach themselves to antithrombin III molecules. This results in a configurational change in antithrombin III molecules so they can rapidly form complexes with the activated serine proteases of the intrinsic pathway and thus delay the coagulation process. Almost all coagulation tests may be affected by heparin. These include the whole-blood clotting time, the activated partial thromboplastin time, the thromboplastin generation test, the prothrombin time, the thombin time, and specific coagulation factor assays based on these tests.

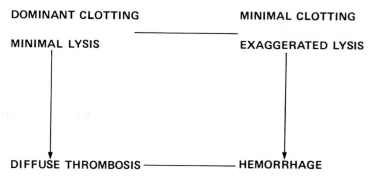

Figure 2-5.   Relationships between thrombosis and hemorrhage in DIC.

TABLE 2-9. Expected Laboratory Results in Various Stages of DIC

	Decompensated	Compensated	Over-Compensated
Platelet count	↓ (< 100,000)	N or ↓	N
Thrombin time	↑ + +	↑ ±	↑ + or ±
Fibrinogen level	↓	N	↑
FDPs	↑ + +	↑ +	↑ +
P.T.	↑	N	N
APTT	↑	N	↓
3P, ethanol gel	+	±	±
Dx	Established DIC ? present, past, continuing*	Mild, chronic Process ?continuing*	Recovery from DIC Early DIC*

* Needs sequential testing

Heparin has been used extensively in the treatment of thromboembolic conditions; and when administered therapeutically, it acts as described above. The commercial product is prepared from beef lung or intestinal mucosa and is usually administered subcutaneously or intravenously. The whole-blood clotting time was traditionally used to monitor the anticoagulant effects of heparin; however, the activated partial thromboplastin time is much more practical and, if used properly, more accurate in monitoring heparin's anticoagulant effect. The correlation is least good when the anticoagulant activity is greatest. The type of APTT reagent used is of prime importance because some reagents are more sensitive than others to the heparin effect.

When heparin is administered by continuous infusion, the anticoagulant effect should be tested soon after initiation of therapy and at least once daily, preferably at the same time each day. Individual patients vary in their responsiveness to the drug, and requirements may change from day to day. When heparin is administered intermittently by the intravenous route, the testing should be done just before the next dose is to be given in order to determine whether evidence of the anticoagulant effect is still present. By this method, a proper dose can be selected to produce continuous,

TABLE 2-10. Laboratory Measures of DIC

I. Most Specific and Sensitive Tests
    Paracoagulation (SP)
    FDP
    Fibrinopeptide A
    Serial fibrinogen concentrations

II. Less Specific and Sensitive Tests
    Pro-Time
    APTT
    Thrombin time
    Serial platelet counts

III. Least Specific and Sensitive Tests
    Euglobulin clot lysis
    Factor assays other than fibrinogen
    Peripheral blood smear

although variable, anticoagulant activity. After this is accomplished, one needs to perform such testing only once daily. When subcutaneous low-dose heparin is given for prophylactic reasons, there is rarely any need to monitor therapy, since, when given in the proper dosage, no significant change occurs in coagulation tests. It is important to remember that so long as a significant concentration of heparin is present, it is impossible to evaluate coagulation studies except in reference to the effect of heparin. Thus, a prothrombin time performed in the presence of circulating heparin does not give specific information concerning the effects of coumarin-type anticoagulants. Heparin can cause thrombocytopenia, probably on an immunologic basis. This usually occurs after 4 to 7 days of treatment; and for this reason, patients receiving heparin therapy should have periodic platelet counts.

As with oral anticoagulant therapy, hemorrhage is the most common complication of heparin therapy. Careful laboratory monitoring of its effect may help to reduce such problems. Factitious administration of heparin has been reported in health-related personnel and may pose a difficult diagnostic problem.

When streptokinase and urokinase are used in the treatment of thrombotic disorders, the effect is to produce systemic fibrinogenolysis as well as local fibrinolysis by the activation of plasminogen to plasmin. The result is an increased rate of clot lysis and prolongation of all of the whole blood and plasma clotting tests. It is important to perform at least one test such as the activated partial thromboplastin time or thrombin time to ensure that the fibrinolytic state is achieved. When therapy is to be discontinued and heparin therapy is to be started, it is necessary to measure the fibrinogen level, which should be greater than 100 mg% before the initial dose of heparin is given. Hemorrhage is an even greater problem with the use of these enzymes than with oral anticoagulants and heparin.

Because of their effect on platelet function, drugs such as aspirin are frequently used as antithrombotic agents. Aspirin may cause gastric bleeding after prolonged use and may increase the bleeding time, but its main importance is its effect on the platelet release reaction, which causes an abnormality in platelet aggregation with most commonly used aggregating agents. This effect of aspirin on platelet function continues as long as a platelet survives, which may be as long as 10 days, but new platelets released in the absence of aspirin function normally. Thus the degree of the demonstrable effect depends on the time of aspirin ingestion with relation to the time of testing. Many other drugs, particularly other nonsteroidal anti-inflammatory drugs, produce similar effects on the release reaction and aggregation of platelets, but the effect is often milder and only present while an effective level of the drug is in the circulation. Dipyridamole does not effect aggregation but has been shown to increase platelet survival in patients with shortened survival prior to therapy. Dextran is also sometimes administered intravenously for its antithrombotic effect.

References

Bick RL: Alterations of hemostasis associated with malignancy: etiology, pathophysiology, diagnosis and management. Semin Thromb Hemostas 5:1, 1978.

Bick RL: Alterations of hemostasis associated with cardiopulmonary bypass: pathophysiology, prevention, diagnosis and management. Semin Thromb Hemostas 3:59, 1976.

Deykin D: Antithrombotic therapy, rationale and application. Postgrad Med 65:135, 1979.

Fekete LF, and Bick RL: Laboratory modalities for assessing hemostasis during cardiopulmonary bypass. Semin Thromb Hemostas 3:83, 1976.

Hirsch J: Hypercoagulability. Semin Hematol *14:*409, 1977.

Israel MCG, and Delamore IW (eds): Hematologic Aspects of Systemic Disease. Clin Haematol *1*(3):445, 1972.

Kelton JG, and Hirsch J: Bleeding associated with antithrombotic therapy. Semin Hematol *17:*259, 1980.

Schmaier AH, et al: Factitious heparin administration. Ann Intern Med *95:*592, 1981.

Sirridge MS, et al: Effects of antiplatelet drugs on platelet function tests. Mo Med *96:*212, 1979.

Sirridge MS: Disseminated intravascular coagulation: a practical approach to its diagnosis. J Kan Med Soc *71:*378, 1970.

Spero JA, Lewis JH, and Haseba U: Disseminated intravascular coagulation: findings in 346 patients. Thromb Haemost *43:*28, 1980.

Thal AP, et al: Shock, A Physiologic Basis for Treatment. Chicago, Year Book Medical Publishers, 1971.

CHAPTER *3*

General Principles of Testing

COLLECTION OF BLOOD

Venous Blood

Blood should be drawn as rapidly as possible and placed without delay into an anticoagulant. With a good, clean venipuncture, it is possible to use a vacuum tube system to draw samples for most hemostatic testing. For some tests, however, it is important that samples not be contaminated with tissue factors, and for this reason, the two-syringe technique is preferable for them.

A hemostasis work-up may include both a coagulopathy study and a platelet function study. Such studies require as much as 30 to 40 ml of blood. To obtain and to dispense this amount of blood before it clots is sometimes difficult. Therefore, we make use of a two-syringe technique, using Vacutainer (Becton-Dickinson, B-D) tubes and one plastic syringe. Figure 3-1 shows a way in which blood may be drawn and distributed for such a hemostasis work-up. A special Luer (BD) adaptor, which fits into the hub of a standard needle, is attached to a collecting Vacutainer holder and used for initial venipuncuture. After venipuncture, this system is cleansed of tissue thromboplastin by first drawing blood into a red-stoppered Vacutainer tube. This sample may be used for any test requiring serum, or it may be discarded. Samples for the tests requiring plasma are drawn next, thus taking advantage of a two-syringe technique. After the Vacutainer tubes containing citrate anticoagulant are filled, the Vacutainer holder, with the Luer adaptor still attached, is removed and a plastic syringe is attached to the needle. In this syringe, 20 ml of blood is drawn for additional platelet function tests. Heparin can be added to ten ml of this blood for testing of platelet retention, and the remainder of the blood used for the quantitative clot-retraction test. With this system, anticoagulation of the samples is immediate, which avoids the likelihood of clotted samples.

Capillary Blood

Occasionally, it may be difficult to obtain venous blood from a patient. Because of the greater ease of obtaining capillary blood from infants, one is tempted to use such blood for coagulation procedures. Capillary blood can be used for some procedures,

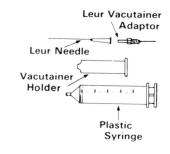

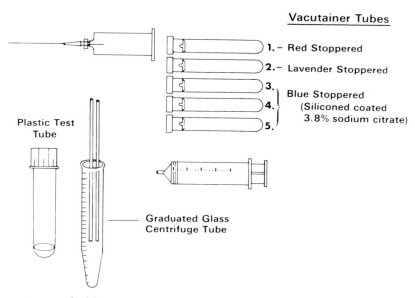

Figure 3-1.   **Method for drawing and distributing blood for a complete hemostasis work-up.**

provided it is obtained rapidly and anticoagulated immediately. The Miale Pro-thrombin Pipet (Dade), which contains oxalate, can be used for obtaining capillary blood for the prothrombin time (PT), but is not satisfactory for other tests.

ANTICOAGULANTS

Although both oxalate and citrate are satisfactory anticoagulants for coagulation tests, citrate is preferred; it gives better preservation of factors V and VIII. Citrated samples are also more sensitive to the presence of heparin and, therefore, are pre-ferred for tests used in monitoring heparin therapy. When oxalate binds with cal-cium, insoluble complexes or precipitates are formed that may interfere with end-point detection in automated clotting systems with photo-optical end points. At least one-half hour should elapse between collection of the sample and the time of testing, when citrate is used.

Blood for coagulation studies is usually drawn in the ratio of 1 part anticoagulant to 9 parts of whole blood. A 3.8% solution of the anticoagulant sodium citrate is probably the most widely used concentration. Under most conditions this concentration is satisfactory, but when hematocrit values exceed 50%, as in polycythemias and in the newborn, the quantity of calcium in the decreased plasma volume is not enough to completely bind the citrate and spurious prolongation of prothrombin time (PT) and activated partial thromboplastin time (APTT) may occur. To avoid this problem, the ratio of blood to anticoagulant should be adjusted, based on the patient's hematocrit value. Studies have shown that probably only half the concentration of 3.8% citrate is required to anticoagulate normal blood samples. The use of a lower concentration, such as 3.2%, has no apparent effect on test values from patients with low hematocrits. Therefore, it is possible to routinely use lower concentrations of citrate, and thus avoid problems in testing samples from patients with high hematocrit values. The 3.2% concentration has been adopted as the standard for coagulation studies by the International Committee for Standardization in Hematology. Acid citrate buffered to a lower pH is preferred by some laboratories and is contained in the new Vacutainer Coag Tubes (B-D).

Heparin should not be used as an anticoagulant for collecting blood samples for coagulation studies. It acts with antithrombin III and inhibits many of the coagulation reactions. Heparin is the anticoagulant of choice, however, when collecting blood for platelet-retention studies.

Ethylenediaminetetraacetic acid (EDTA) is not a satisfactory anticoagulant for blood that is to be used in coagulation tests. It is believed to inhibit or interfere with the polymerization of fibrinogen in the formation of the fibrin clot, and factor V is unstable in its presence. It is, however, the anticoagulant of choice for the isolation and examination of platelets.

CENTRIFUGATION

To obtain platelet-rich plasma (PRP), anticoagulated blood is centrifuged for 10 minutes at 1000 rpm. Plasma should be removed immediately with a plastic or siliconized pipette and stored in stoppered plastic or siliconized tubes. This plasma may be used for platelet-aggregation studies and the direct method for platelet-factor-3 (PF_3) availability.

To obtain platelet-poor plasma (PPP), anticoagulated blood is centrifuged for 10 minutes at 3000 rpm. Plasma should be removed immediately and placed in stoppered plastic or siliconized tubes. This plasma may be used for most coagulation testing.

For some tests, such as β-thromboglobulin (B-TG) and platelet factor 4 (PF_4), centrifugation of samples should take place at a temperature of 2 to 4°C. For this process, a refrigerated centrifuge is required.

HOLDING SAMPLES FOR TESTING

Once blood is drawn, changes begin to occur. The early surface reactions do not require calcium, so they occur in anticoagulated samples. Labile factors such as V and VIII may become inactive. Platelets are sufficiently altered in 3 hours that platelet function testing is unsatisfactory. Plastic or siliconized test tubes are recommended for both collecting and handling samples for most tests. Glass Vacutainers (B-D) can be used for the prothrombin time (PT) and activated partial thromboplastin time (APTT), but if such tests are not to be done immediately, samples should remain in unopened tubes at room temperature. The plasma from centrifuged samples should be stored at 4°C for a time not to exceed 2 hours. Changes in the sample within this period of time are usually minimal and of little or no clinical significance. Blood drawn for platelet-function studies should remain at room temperature, and it should be processed immediately after drawing. The testing of these samples should not exceed 3 hours.

If plasma is to be frozen, it must be done rapidly at $-20°C$ or lower. Slow freezing may denature the clotting proteins. When a frozen sample is to be used for testing, it must be rapidly thawed at 37° C to prevent denaturation of fibrinogen.

TEMPERATURE

All biologic reagents and all plasma and blood samples, except those to be used for platelet function studies, should be kept in the refrigerator or in an ice bath until time for testing. All clotting procedures should be carried out at 37°C, using a constant-temperature water bath or heating block.

INFLUENCE OF TIME

The instability of reagents and of blood and plasma samples tends to cause a bias in results that is related to the time involved in making repeated determinations. For this reason, it is often necessary to obtain a control specimen at the same time and under the same conditions that the patient's sample is obtained. These two specimens can be checked repeatedly against each other throughout the period of testing. When substitutions are being made in such time-consuming procedures as the thromboplastin-generation test, it is wise to rerun the patient's own sample at the end of the period of testing to detect possible changes that may have occurred during the time interval of testing. Blood specimens that are deficient in the factors involved in contact activation (factors XII, XI, prekallikrein, HMWK) are particularly likely to show improved coagulability on standing, especially when stored in glass test tubes. Random order should be utilized when multiple samples are being tested at one time.

TYPES OF TESTS

Clotting End Point

Clotting end-point tests measure the multienzyme reactions involved in clotting by the detection of a fibrin clot and are of three general types: (1) those based on the clotting time of whole blood or plasma, (2) those based on the indirect prothrombin consumption methods, (3) two-stage methods in which a coagulant is formed in one tube and its potency assayed on a substrate in another tube. The appearance of the clot that is formed depends to some extent on the rate of clotting. For this reason, it becomes increasingly difficult to pinpoint the exact moment of clotting as the time becomes extended. Examples are clots formed in prolonged PT and APTT tests and the assay procedures that involve increasing dilutions of plasma. Frequently, the period from the first appearance of strands of fibrin to the actual formation of a solid clot may extend for several seconds. We have elected to wait for the formation of a visible web of fibrin strands in such procedures and to call this the end point. When plasma clots rapidly, one is unable to see the strand and web formation, as the change from liquid to solid occurs within a second. With manual methods, a good light source and a black background make it easier to see the end point; a magnifying glass may also be helpful.

Extended or prolonged clotting times also pose problems when automated instruments employing photo-optical systems are used. The rate of clotting may be so slow and the formed clot of such poor quality that the instrument does not detect the clot and fails to deactivate or stop the timer. When this happens, the clotting time appears to be more prolonged than it really is. Therefore, laboratories should routinely establish a point at which all prolonged values are rechecked with a visual examination of clot formation.

In most clotting end-point methodology, the measurement of time is the basic diagnostic parameter. Some clotting techniques have shown that time alone does not necessarily present a complete profile of coagulation and hemostasis. The levels of clotting factors may be reduced, and this may not be reflected by prolonged clotting times. The clot may form in a normal period of time, but in an abnormal manner. For this reason, instruments that reflect the dynamics or kinetics of fibrin formation are opening new areas in coagulation investigation. The Bio-Data Coagulation profiler is such an instrument, and it provides a tracing that is referred to as a thrombokinetogram. We use this instrument in our laboratory.

Synthetic Substrate

Direct, quantitative measures of some of the clotting enzymes can be achieved by measuring the proteolysis of synthetically prepared substrates. A synthetic substrate duplicates that part of the amino acid sequence of its natural counterpart at which the activated split by a proteolytic enzyme occurs. Some synthetic substrates are more specific than others, but there are satisfactory substrates for measuring the proteolytic activity of thrombin, factor X, plasmin, kallikrein, urokinase, and others. The chromogenic substrates are oligopeptide p-nitroanalides, and the end point when they are used is color development, which is measured by a spectrophotometer. The fluorogenic substrates are similar in structure but contain a detecting fluorophase group, and the end point is the development of fluorescence, which can be detected by a fluorometer. Enzyme instability, formation of fibrin strands, and turbidity may contribute to difficulties in detecting such end points.

Immunologic

The precise quantitation of some proteolytic enzymes can be done by the technique of radial immunodiffusion (RID). A protein antigen is applied to a well in a thin gel media containing a monospecific antigen. The antigen-antibody complexes diffuse radially, forming a zone of precipitation around the well. The diameter of this precipitation zone is proportional to the concentration of the antigen and is compared to a specific standard for quantitation.

Electroimmunodiffusion (EID) utilizes the principles of RID, but adds the forces of electrophoresis, which causes the antigen to move into the antibody media. The results of the movement of such antigen-antibody complexes is a spike or rocket. The peak height of the rocket is directly proportional to the concentration of the antigen. Crossed immunoelectrophoresis is another modification that is used in the diagnosis of von Willebrand's disease.

Direct measurement of proteolytic enzymes may also be accomplished by the radioimmunoassay technique (RIA). RIA is dependent on the competition between the naturally occurring proteolytic enzyme in a sample and added isotope-labeled enzyme for a limited number of binding sites on a specific antibody to that enzyme. The radioactivity of the bound material is measured in a gamma counter. The amount of the isotope-labeled enzyme bound by the antibody is inversely proportional to the concentration of unlabeled enzyme present. Such tests can only measure immunoreactive proteins and not their coagulant activity.

METHODOLOGY

Appropriate methodology must be used in coagulation testing or meaningful results will not be obtained. Deviations from manufacturer's instructions in the performance of tests should be avoided, unless the laboratory has done extensive testing with an altered technique. The incubation time of activation mixtures, such as in the APTT, should be carried out as recommended. Whereas some APTT reagents will give approximately the same clotting time with various incubation times, others will show significant changes in values, which can lead to false interpretation. This point becomes important in the case of some of the contact-factor deficiencies in which increased activation time may cause shortening of the APTT. We prefer the 5-minute incubation time.

Considerable variation exists in reagents that are marketed for use in a single test. This is particularly true of APTT reagents. Those which utilize ellagic acid as an activator may fail to detect a deficiency of prekallikrein. The significant variation in the detection of heparin effect among such reagents makes it necessary for each laboratory to construct a curve, adding known amounts of heparin to a plasma pool in order to determine the sensitivity of the system being used. Buffered reagents are helpful in minimizing such variations. It is advisable to use controls furnished by the manufacturer of reagents selected.

SCREENING TESTS

No single screening test can determine the adequacy of hemostatic function. The use of the routine bleeding time and clotting time is to be condemned, as is the use of the partial thromboplastin time as an isolated screening procedure. The following approach, although far from simple, offers the best type of screening for all aspects of the hemostatic mechanism when this is required.

1. Platelet estimation to evaluate platelet numbers.
2. Bleeding time to test in vivo vascular and platelet functions in primary hemostasis.
3. PT to evaluate the extrinsic pathway.
4. APTT to evaluate the intrinsic pathway.
5. Clot retraction to evaluate platelets and fibrinogen and to examine the character of the whole-blood clot.

FOLLOW-UP TESTING

If abnormalities are detected through the screening tests, further studies may be conducted according to the following suggested outline.

1. If platelet numbers are decreased, the bleeding time, tourniquet test, clot retraction, and prothrombin consumption test may show abnormal reactions but are usually not helpful in diagnosis or therapy.

2. If bleeding time is prolonged, some or all of the following tests should be performed.
   a. Tourniquet test.
   b. Platelet count.
   c. Evaluation of platelet morphology and clumping on a peripheral smear made from blood that has not been mixed with anticoagulants.
   d. Platelet function tests:
      (1) Quantitative clot retraction.
      (2) In vivo platelet adhesiveness or in vitro platelet retention in glass bead columns.
      (3) Platelet aggregation tests, including ristocetin aggregation.
      (4) Prothrombin consumption test.
      (5) Platelet-factor-3 availability test.
   e. Activated partial thromboplastin time and possibly, factor VIII level.

3. If the APTT is prolonged and the PT is normal, the following may be helpful.
   a. Repeat the APTT on a new sample and possibly test the sample with a different APTT reagent. If prolongation is confirmed, repeat with 10-and 20-minute incubation times.
   b. If prolonged incubation does not correct the abnormality, mix equal parts of patient's plasma and control plasma and repeat the test.
   c. If correction by the control plasma is incomplete, do further testing for a circulating anticoagulant.
   d. If mixture with control plasma corrects the abnormal result, the differential APTT may be helpful.
   e. Do specific assays for factors VIII, IX, or the contact factors as indicated by history or the differential APTT.

4. If the PT is prolonged and the APTT is normal, the following may be helpful.
   a. Repeat the PT on a new sample, and if prolongation is confirmed, proceed to b.
   b. Mix equal parts of patient's plasma and control plasma and repeat the test.
   c. If correction by the control plasma is incomplete, do further testing for a circulating anticoagulant.
   d. If control plasma corrects the abnormal result, a factor VII deficiency is the most likely cause.
   e. The PT with Simplastin A, Stypven time, and thrombin time may also be of some differential value.
   f. Do specific assays for factors I, II, V, VII, or X as indicated by the history or by these tests.

5. If both the APTT and the PT are prolonged, the following may be helpful.
   a. Repeat the tests on a new sample, and if prolongation is confirmed, proceed to b.
   b. Mix equal parts of the patient's plasma and control plasma and repeat both tests.
   c. If correction by the control plasma is incomplete, do further testing for a circulating anticoagulant.
   d. If control plasma corrects the abnormal result, differential APTT and PT tests may be helpful, especially if a single-factor deficiency is suspected. Multiple deficiencies occur in vitamin K deficiency, oral anticoagulant therapy, and DIC and are more difficult to sort out. Combined inherited deficiencies are also possible.
   e. Assay procedures should be selected as indicated by history and differential tests.
   f. The PT with Simplastin A, Stypven time, and thrombin time may be of some differential value.
6. If clot retraction is abnormal, the following tests may be helpful.
   a. Platelet count or estimation and evaluation of platelet clumping on a peripheral blood smear made from nonanticoagulated blood.
   b. Bleeding time.
   c. Platelet aggregation tests and possibly other platelet function tests.
   d. Thrombin time.
   e. Assay for factor I (fibrinogen), especially if the clot is small and shows increased red cell fallout.
   f. CBC when increased red cell fallout is present, as this may suggest polycythemia vera.
7. If disseminated intravascular coagulation (DIC) is suspected, some or all of these tests should be done.
   a. Platelet count.
   b. Serial fibrinogen levels.
   c. Protamine sulfate or ethanol gelation test for soluble fibrin monomer complexes (SFMC).
   d. Test for fibrin degredation products (FDP) in serum.
   e. Euglobulin clot lysis test.
   f. Serial PT tests may be helpful, especially if the test was prolonged initially.

RELATIONSHIP OF TESTS TO HEMOSTATIC MECHANISM

In Figure 3-2, the important hemostatic tests are superimposed on a diagram of the scheme of the hemostatic mechanism in order to indicate which functions and reactions are evaluated by each test. The accompanying list gives further details concerning the diagnostic value of the tests.
1. Tourniquet test measures the ability of small blood vessels to retain red cells under conditions of stress or trauma. The reaction is most often positive in vascular disorders, thrombocytopenia, platelet functional defects and disorders of fibrinogen.

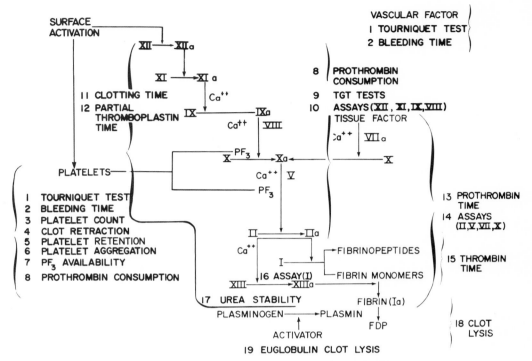

Figure 3-2.   Relationships of hemostatic tests to the hemostatic mechanism.

2. Bleeding time is a measurement of primary hemostasis, the time required for bleeding to stop after injury to superficial small blood vessels. It may be prolonged in vascular disorders, thrombocytopenia, functional platelet abnormalities, after the ingestion of aspirin and related drugs, and in disorders of fibrinogen.

3. Platelets are present in normal numbers in all conditions except primary or secondary thrombocytopenia. Moderate to marked reduction in platelet count usually occurs in acute DIC.

4. Clot retraction is dependent on (a) platelet numbers and the functional capacity of the platelets, (b) the quantity of fibrinogen, and (c) the packed cell volume. Retraction and expression of serum from the clot are poor in thrombocytopenia. The clot is small, and red cell fallout is increased with fibrinogenopenia and abnormalities of fibrinogen. An increased packed cell volume usually results in increased red cell fallout, as in polycythemia.

5. Platelet retention (adhesiveness) is a measure of the ability of platelets to adhere to foreign surfaces. Platelet retention in vivo may be estimated by comparing the platelet count in anticoagulated venous blood to that in capillary blood collected at regular intervals after a small skin incision is made. In vitro retention may be tested by comparing platelet counts in venous blood before and after exposure to glass bead columns. The per-

centage of retention of platelets is calculated. Platelet retention is diminished in von Willebrand's disease and some other disorders of platelet function.

6. Platelet aggregation is a measure of the ability of platelets to adhere to each other and to form aggregates. Platelet aggregation may be studied by determining the changes in light transmission through platelet-rich plasma as platelets aggregate and disaggregate in response to various stimuli such as ADP, epinephrine, thrombin, collagen, and ristocetin. As platelets aggregate, there is a decrease in optical density of the platelet-rich plasma that can be recorded continuously in an aggregometer. Defects in platelet aggregation may be inherited but are more commonly acquired, as in ingestion of certain drugs (especially aspirin), renal failure, liver disease, and fibrinolytic states.

7. Platelet-factor-3 (PF_3) availability tests measure the reaction in which phospholipid (PF_3) is made available on platelet surfaces during the coagulation process. One way in which this can be measured is by determining changes in the Kaolin clotting time of platelet-rich plasma over time. Also, a single measurement can be made by doing a recalcification time on a plasma sample, containing a known number of platelets (50,000 per ml), which has been incubated with kaolin and adrenalin. Isolated deficiency of PF_3 is not known to occur, but conditions in which platelets fail to make phospholipid available normally are some of the inherited platelet function defects and various acquired conditions such as uremia, serum protein abnormalities, and ingestion of some drugs.

8. Prothrombin consumption is a method that compares the prothrombin time of serum with that of plasma, thus measuring the consumption of prothrombin during the coagulation process, and indirectly, the intrinsic formation of the prothrombin converting complex. The test is nonspecific, but the findings are often abnormal with thrombocytopenia, platelet function defects, moderate to marked deficiencies of the contact factors (XII, XI, prekallikrein, and high molecular weight kininogen), factors VIII, IX and X, and with some types of circulating anticoagulants.

9. Thromboplastin generation tests (TGT) are two-stage tests that directly measure the amount of prothrombin converting complex that is generated via the intrinsic pathway. Such tests are used primarily to test for deficiencies of the contact factors and factors VIII and IX. Abnormalities in platelet function may be detected if actual suspensions of platelets from patients are used rather than a platelet substitute. Some types of circulating anticoagulants, particularly those specifically active against factor VIII, also cause abnormal results.

10. Assays for the contact factors and factors VIII and IX utilize the activated partial thromboplastin time as a one-stage method for measuring the levels of these factors in plasma. The factor VIII assay is particularly indicated in the diagnosis of von Willebrand's disease, as the level of this factor may be only slightly reduced in the condition. Assays of factors VIII and IX are particularly important in the diagnosis of hemophilia of moderate to mild

severity in which other tests may not be diagnostic. They are necessary to determine exact factor levels in patients and levels attained with infused plasma and factor concentrates.

11. Clotting time is a simple overall test of the intrinsic pathway and may be prolonged by deficiency of any of the clotting factors except VII and XIII. The test lacks sensitivity and specificity and usually is only affected by significant deficiencies; however, almost all circulating anticoagulants produce significant prolongation of the clotting time. The clotting time should not be used as a primary screening test because there are better tests of equal simplicity.

12. Activated partial thromboplastin time (APTT) is a sensitive indicator of deficiencies of all clotting factors except factors VII and XIII. It is a measure of the rate of clotting by the intrinsic pathway and is particularly sensitive to moderate deficiencies of factors VIII and IX. One-stage assay procedures for the contact factors and factors VIII and IX utilize the APTT. The test is affected by heparin and may be used to monitor heparin therapy. Circulating anticoagulants produce prolongation, and the test may be utilized in mixing procedures for detection and assay of anticoagulant activity.

13. Prothrombin time (PT) measures the clotting of plasma with tissue thromboplastin and is prolonged with deficiencies of factors VII, V, and X. Low levels of factor II (prothrombin) and factor I (fibrinogen) affect the test as well. Some types of circulating anticoagulants also produce prolongation. Assay procedures for factors VII, X, V, and II utilize the PT. The PT is used to monitor therapy with oral anticoagulants.

14. Assays of factors II, V, VII, and X utilize the PT as a method of measuring the individual factor levels quantitatively. These values may be decreased in both inherited and acquired deficiencies. Acquired deficiencies are usually multiple.

15. Thrombin time measures the time required for a standard thrombin solution to convert factor I (fibrinogen) in plasma to factor Ia (fibrin). It is influenced by the quantity and quality of fibrinogen present in the plasma and also by the presence of inhibitory substances that interfere with the thrombin-fibrinogen reaction. It is prolonged in the presence of hypofibrinogenemia, dysfibrinogenemia, heparin, fibrinogen-fibrin degradation products (FDP), and abnormal serum proteins (as in multiple myeloma).

16. Assay of factor I (fibrinogen) measures the actual quantity of this protein present in plasma. In afibrinogenemia, the factor is completely absent. It is variably decreased in inherited and acquired fibrinogenopenic states. Inherited and acquired dysfibrinogenemias also occur.

17. Urea stability is a qualitative test that measures the stable cross-linked form of fibrin. Factor XIII (fibrin-stabilizing factor) is necessary for the formation of a clot that is stable in 5M urea or 1% monochloroacetic acid. Defective crossed linkage of fibrin is found in severe inherited and acquired deficiencies of factor XIII.

18. Clot lysis tests measure the overall fibrinolytic activity of blood. Increased

fibrinolysis may be demonstrated in a variety of clinical situations and may be associated with DIC and some liver diseases.

19. Euglobulin clot lysis measures overall fibrinolysis but is especially sensitive to increased quantities of the activator of plasminogen. This test is particularly useful in patients whose blood is incoagulable because of the administration of heparin for cardiac surgery procedures, since in this test the euglobulin fraction of plasma is separated from inhibitors, including heparin, and then later clotted with thrombin. Also, the procedure can be completed in a relatively short time.

References

Beck W: Determination of antisera titres using the single radial immuno-diffusion method. Immunochemistry 6:539, 1969.

Hathaway WE, and Alsever J: The relations of "Fletcher factor" to factors XI and XII. Br J Haematol 18:164, 1970.

Hattersley PG, and Hayse D: The effect of increased contact activation time on the activated partial thromboplastin time. Am J Clin Pathol 16:479, 1976.

Koepke JA, Rodgers JL, and Ollivier MJ: Preinstrumental variables in coagulation testing. Am J Clin Pathol 64:591, 1975.

Laurell CB: Quantitative estimation of proteins by electrophoresis in agarose gel containing antibodies. Anal Biochem 15:45, 1966.

Odegard OR, Lie M, and Abildgaard U: Heparin cofactor activity measured with an amidolytic method. Thromb Res 6:287, 1975.

Shapiro MD, Huntzinger SW, and Wilson JE: Variation among commercial activated partial thromboplastin time reagents in response to heparin. Am J Clin Plathol 67:480, 1977.

CHAPTER *4*

Evaluation of the Vascular Factor

TOURNIQUET TEST

General Principles

The least scientific of the hemorrhagic studies are those used to evaluate the adequacy of blood vessels in the maintenance of normal hemostasis. Capillary fragility procedures (i.e., tourniquet tests) are tests of the ability of the small blood vessels to retain red cells under conditions of stress or trauma and are influenced not only by the vessels themselves but also by platelets. The most commonly used tests are those utilizing positive pressure from a blood pressure cuff. The cuff retards venous return, thus producing hypoxia and conditions of increased pressure in vessels. There is little standardization of such procedures, and all normal persons will have a positive reaction if the pressure is maintained at a high level for a long time. A small percentage of apparently normal persons may have a few petechiae after the usual performance of the test, but the reaction is most often positive in thrombocytopenia, fibrinogenopenia, and vascular purpura. It is usually negative in the hemophilioid states.

Procedure

Carefully inspect the arm for pre-existing petechiae. Apply a blood pressure cuff and determine the blood pressure. Then maintain the pressure halfway between diastolic and systolic with a maximal value of 100 mm Hg for 5 minutes. Release the cuff and observe the arm for several minutes. If petechiae appear during the time the pressure is being applied, release the cuff immediately and consider the reaction positive.

If this test is being done in conjunction with a bleeding time test, the bleeding time procedure should be performed first. If petechiae appear during the time the cuff is being maintained at 40 mm Hg, then the reaction may be reported as positive, and no further testing need be done. If, however, the bleeding time is completed and is normal without the appearance of petechiae, the pressure should then be increased to a level half-way between diastolic and systolic and maintained there for an additional 5 minutes. The reaction may be reported as negative or from 1 to 4 plus,

70

depending on the number of petechiae that appear. An alternate method of reporting is to count the number of petechiae in a stated area.

Normal Value

Normally the reaction is negative.

Reference

Miller SE, (ed): A Textbook of Clinical Pathology, 7th Ed. Baltimore, Williams & Wilkins, 1966, p. 148.

BLEEDING TIME

General Principles

The bleeding time measures the ability to seal off a small wound. It is to some extent dependent on the thickness and vascularity of the skin and on the site of the wound. The puncture must be adequate to produce a free flow of blood (drops at least 0.5 mm in diameter). Skin temperature is important, as vasoconstriction in a cold room may prevent any active bleeding from a small wound. In many patients, the first drops are small because of reflex vasoconstriction. The bleeding time from two puncture wounds may differ significantly; if the difference is too great, the test should be repeated on the other arm. Usually, however, the longest time is considered the most significant. The end point may not be definite because of prolonged oozing of blood-tinged fluid. This oozing occurs in normal persons, as well as in patients with hemorrhagic disease, and therefore should probably be ignored (the time at which free bleeding ceases should be taken as the end point). Occasionally, a small hematoma forms at the puncture site, and this should be reported, as it may indicate increased vascular fragility or abnormality of the supportive tissues.

A prolonged bleeding time is probably always significant. Unfortunately, some patients with bleeding-time abnormalities show a variation in the test results from one time to another, and the bleeding time may sometimes be found to be completely normal. Before the regular use of the template bleeding-time technique, it was assumed that the bleeding time might not always be abnormal in disorders of primary hemostasis and that prolonged bleeding times were rarely found in the absence of disease. The template procedure offers greater sensitivity and is influenced significantly by the ingestion of aspirin and similar medications. In the absence of drug ingestion, a prolonged template bleeding time should still be considered as evidence of some abnormality of hemostasis.

To some extent, the bleeding time measures the adequacy of small blood vessels, but it is also influenced by the ability of platelets to form hemostatic plugs in these vessels. Most techniques utilize a blood pressure cuff to produce some venous stasis in order to stress the local hemostatic mechanism. The bleeding time may be prolonged in diseases that affect the ability of the vessels to constrict and retract and in diseases in which there is a decrease in platelet numbers (thrombocytopenia) or a defect in platelet function. It is important to question the patient carefully concerning drug intake during a period of several days prior to the time of testing. Aspirin prolongs the bleeding time by a few minutes in most subjects, but this effect is much more marked in patients with von Willebrand's disease and platelet function defects. Also, the combination of aspirin and alcohol ingestion has been reported to prolong the bleeding time more than aspirin alone; although alcohol alone has no effect. Corticosteroids may shorten the bleeding time in patients with some defects of primary hemostasis but not in von Willebrand's disease. With the exception of abnormalities of fibrinogen, disorders of coagulation are rarely associated with prolongation of bleeding time, but recurrent, delayed bleeding may occur later at the incision site if the clotting mechanism is ineffective. In addition, ingestion of aspirin by patients with hemophilia may cause significant prolongation of the bleeding time, particularly when the template method is used.

Ivy Method Procedure

The blood pressure cuff is placed around the arm above the elbow and inflated to 40 mm Hg. This pressure is maintained throughout the procedure. Temperature in the room should be average to avoid either surface vasodilatation or vasoconstriction. The skin of the volar surface of the forearm should be cleaned with alcohol and allowed to dry. It may be necessary to lightly shave the forearm in a few patients with hairy growth. In an area where the skin is held tensed and tightly stretched, two puncture wounds of approximately 3 mm in depth are made with a disposable lancet, care being taken to avoid superficial veins. (It is easy to tell when a vein has been cut because bleeding begins immediately and may be fairly profuse.) A stopwatch is started, and drops of blood are carefully blotted with a filter paper at 30-second intervals so as not to exert pressure on the wound. This procedure is continued until the flow of blood ceases. The bleeding time for both puncture wounds should be recorded. The test should be discontinued at the end of 15 minutes in persons who show no evidence of cessation of bleeding. A pressure bandage should then be applied at the puncture sites.

Normal Value: Mean 3.5 minutes (range 2 to 6 minutes). Values between 6 and 10 minutes have been reported in less than 1% of persons who appear to be normal (Figure 4-1).

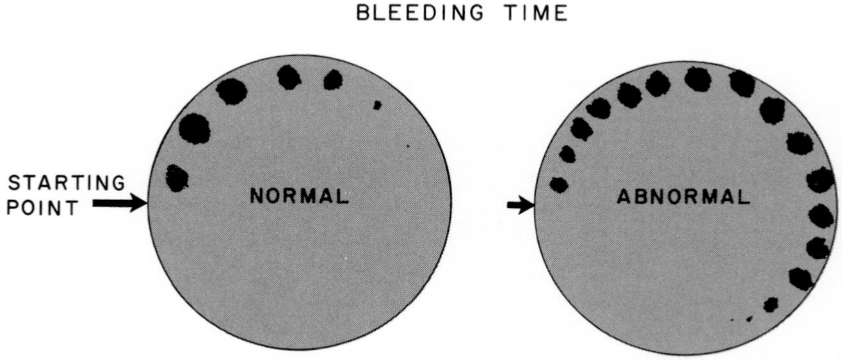

BLEEDING TIME

Figure 4-1.   Ivy bleeding time. Examples of filter paper used to determine the bleeding time in a normal and an abnormal patient.

References

Ivy AC, Shapiro PR, and Melnick P: The bleeding tendency in jaundice. Surg Gynecol Obstet 60:781, 1935.
Miller SE (ed): A Textbook of Clinical Pathology, 7th Ed. Baltimore, Williams & Wilkins, 1966, p. 145.

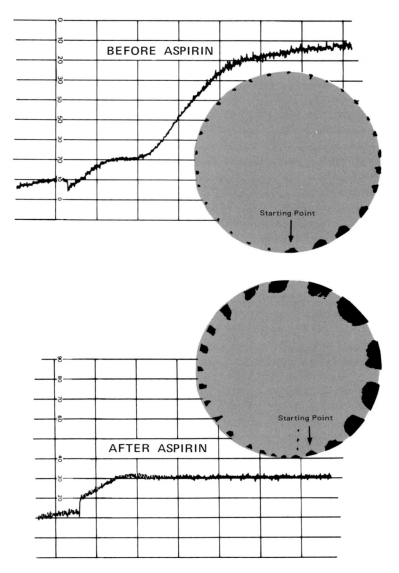

Figure 4-2. Examples of filter paper used to determine the Ivy bleeding time and tracings of platelet aggregation with weak ADP in a patient with a platelet functional defect before and after the administration of aspirin.

Template Method Procedure

Borchgrevink suggested that in vivo platelet adhesiveness could be tested for by comparing the platelet count done on anticoagulated venous blood with blood obtained from an incision 10 mm long and 1 mm in depth made on the volar surface of the forearm. Since this type of cut gives a somewhat longer bleeding time in normal persons, it has been utilized by some laboratories in an effort to increase the sensitivity of the bleeding time test to minor disorders. It utilizes the Ivy technique, except for the type of incision. The availability of a simple, disposable device (Simplate or Simplate II) for making the incision has popularized this test. Simplate makes one linear incision 5 mm in length by 1 mm in depth and Simplate II makes two such incisions. Incisions should be made on the lateral aspect of the volar surface of the forearm 5 cm below the elbow. In infants and small children, it is advisable to modify the technique by decreasing the incision size (5 mm by 0.5 mm) and the pressure level maintained by the blood pressure cuff (20 mm for infants weighing less than 1000 g, 25 mm for infants 1000 to 2000 g, and 30 mm for all infants over 2000 g and small children).

The question of whether the incisions should be horizontal or vertical is an important one. Bleeding times in most subjects are longer with horizontal incisions and prolonged times may be found in normal subjects when this technique is used. It has been suggested that vertical incisions are preferable for routine screening, but that horizontal incisions may be particularly useful in patients who have a history of bleeding. Significant scarring occurs with both, and the use of butterfly adhesive bandages may be helpful. The subject should be informed of the scarring and warned to leave a covering bandage in place for 24 hours after the test is done.

Normal Values: Adults—mean 5 min (range 3 to 10 minutes). Neonates and children (with modified technique)—mean 3 to 5 minutes (range 1 to 6 minutes).

References

Borchgrevink CF: Platelet adhesion in vivo in patients with bleeding disorders. Acta Med Scand *170:*231, 1961.
Borchgrevink CF: A method for measuring platelet adhesiveness in vivo. Acta Med Scand *168:*157, 1960.
Deykin D, Janson P, and McMahon L: Ethanol potentiation of aspirin-induced prolongation of the bleeding time. N Engl J Med *306:*852, 1982.
Feusner JH: Normal and abnormal bleeding time in neonates and young children utilizing a fully standardized template technique. Am J Clin Pathol *74:*73, 1980.
Kumar R, et al: Clinical trial of a new bleeding time device. Am J Clin Pathol *70:*642, 1978.
Mielke CH, et al: The standardized normal Ivy bleeding time and its prolongation by aspirin. Blood *34:*204, 1969.

Aspirin-Tolerance Test Procedure

This bleeding time test is done by any standardized method before and 1 hour after an adult has ingested 5 gr to 10 gr of aspirin. If the initial bleeding time is significantly prolonged, this second test should not be done. The test is also contraindicated in patients with severe hemophilia in whom profoundly prolonged bleeding times may occur after ingestion of aspirin and in whom there may be considerable difficulty in stopping the bleeding.

Normal Value: Using the template method, the mean value after aspirin ingestion is 9½ minutes with a range of 4 minutes to 21 minutes. Drops are frequently larger after aspirin (Figure 4-2).

References

Kameshiro MM, et al: Bleeding time after aspirin in disorders of intrinsic clotting. N Engl J Med *281:*1039, 1969.
Mielke CH, et al: The standardized normal Ivy bleeding time and its prolongation by aspirin. Blood *34:*204, 1969.
Quick AJ: Hemorrhagic Disease and Thrombosis, 2nd Ed. Philadelphia, Lea & Febiger, 1966, p. 386.
Sirridge MS, et al: Effects of antiplatelet drugs on platelet function tests. Mo Med *96:*212, 1979.

CHAPTER *5*

Evaluation of Platelets

The evaluation of platelet numbers may be accomplished by actually counting the platelets after diluting the blood or by examining a stained peripheral blood smear. No platelet count should be reported without examining a smear. Many embarrassing errors can be avoided by taking the small amount of extra time necessary to carry out both procedures.

Direct methods of platelet counting are preferable. Blood collected in EDTA is best because (1) it is more representative of the existing conditions in the circulation, (2) the count can be repeated on the same sample if necessary, and (3) there is no clumping of the platelets, except in cases of hyperaggregability or platelet satellitism, when platelets become adherent to polymorphonuclear neutrophils in vitro.

Adhesiveness, rather than fragility, usually accounts for the loss of platelets. An example of a problem that may be attributed to adhesiveness is that of a patient with petechiae who was studied in our office laboratory and found to have platelet counts of 75,000 and 37,000 when the count was done on blood obtained directly from a finger stick. Unfortunately, the peripheral smear was not studied before the patient was admitted to the hospital. In the hospital, a platelet count made on venous blood collected in EDTA gave a value of 269,000. The peripheral smear showed clumping, which apparently occurred at the site of the puncture and in the pipettes used for diluting the capillary blood obtained from the finger stick. We also studied a patient who had platelet satellitism. The patient was post partum and was suffering from sepsis with a high fever. The in vitro adherence of platelets to neutrophils in blood collected in EDTA was noted on a peripheral smear. A smear made directly from capillary blood did not demonstrate the phenomenon. A platelet count on capillary blood was 181,000, but one done after 4 hours of storage of EDTA blood was 112,000. After 7 hours, the count had decreased to 49,000. The platelets showed increased retention in glass bead columns but normal aggregation. The fibrinogen level was 620%. Treatment with low-molecular-weight dextran resulted in an increase in platelet count to 716,000 and a decrease in glass bead retention.

Platelet adhesiveness is abnormal in many disorders of platelet function. The examples mentioned in the previous paragraph are of in vivo and in vitro adhesiveness, which was discovered accidentally. It is possible to measure in vivo platelet adhesiveness by comparing the platelet count in anticoagulated blood with that obtained from the standardized incision used for the bleeding-time test. It is also possible to measure in vitro platelet adhesiveness to glass beads by comparing the platelet count of normally collected anticoagulated blood with the count in blood that has been exposed to a standardized glass bead column. By both of these methods, platelets have been found to have decreased adhesiveness in von Willebrand's disease, thrombasthenia, some other platelet function defects, myeloid metaplasia, multiple myeloma, macroglobulinemia, severe anemias, and azotemia. Increased adhesiveness has also been reported in a variety of conditions. Platelets seem to have normal adhesiveness in patients suffering from the inherited blood-coagulation disorders.

Other platelet functions may be measured in a variety of ways. The tourniquet test and bleeding time (Chapter 4) measure both platelet and vascular function in primary hemostasis and in protecting small blood vessels under stress. Careful observation of the clot gives information about the clot retraction function and is specifically abnormal in thrombasthenia. The ability of platelets to respond to various aggregating agents can be measured in vitro by testing platelet-rich plasma in an aggregometer. Platelet-factor-3 availability can be measured by the prothrombin consumption test and by incubating platelet-rich plasma with a platelet activator before recalcification. The standard thromboplastin generation test, which is described in Chapter 6, may be used to measure platelet-factor-3 function as well as that of coagulation factors VIII and IX. Variable abnormalities of platelet function are seen in inherited and acquired disorders. It is often possible to specifically characterize these disorders by performing a group of platelet-function tests.

The measurement of circulating platelet aggregates may be helpful in the evaluation of hypercoagulable states. Also, since platelet factor 4 and β-thromboglobulin are released from activated platelets, their measurement in plasma may reflect in vivo activation.

Detection of antibodies that react with platelets is difficult. The available techniques fall into two classifications: those which utilize immunologic reactions and those which are based on the way in which the antibody affects platelet function. Immunologic techniques that can detect and quantify immunoglobulins on platelet surfaces are too complicated for most clinical laboratories and at present remain primarily research procedures. The identification of such antibodies has been useful in proving that most cases of idiopathic thrombocytopenic purpura are of autoimmune etiology. Of all the other techniques, only inhibition of clot retraction is sufficiently rapid and simple to be performed routinely, and this test has been particularly useful in the detection of some drug-related antibodies.

EXAMINATION OF BLOOD SMEAR FOR PLATELET NUMBERS AND MORPHOLOGY

Procedure

1. Smears may be made directly from capillary blood without an anticoagulant or from blood collected in EDTA.
2. In examining smears made from capillary blood, the examiner should first

look at the "fingers" of the smear for clumps of platelets. Unusually large clumps suggest an elevated platelet count, and the absence of any clumps indicates thrombocytopenia. There are usually from 5 to 10 individual platelets plus some clumps in each oil-immersion field.

3. In smears made from blood collected in EDTA, no clumping of platelets occurs, and this valuable parameter for estimating platelet numbers is not applicable. The average number of individual platelets per oil-immersion field is higher (10 to 20) because of the absence of clumping.

4. Abnormalities of size, shape, or granularity should also be noted and reported.

PLATELET COUNTING

Manual Methods

Reagent

The diluting fluid for direct platelet counts may be either ammonium oxalate solution or sodium citrate solution. Ammonium oxalate is used in a 1% concentration. It lakes red blood cells, and is preferable in phase-contrast microscopy. Sodium citrate does not lake red blood cells, and is most often used with ordinary light microscopy. Both ammonium oxalate and sodium citrate solution should be filtered before use to remove artifacts.

Procedure

1. Draw diluting fluid to the 0.5 mark in the red-cell pipette; then draw up either capillary blood or blood collected in EDTA until the column reaches the 1.0 mark, and fill the pipette with diluting fluid to the 101 mark. This provides a 1:200 dilution of the blood. Shake the pipette vigorously. Unopettes (Becton-Dickinson), which contain 1% ammonium oxalate as a diluent in a dilution ratio of 1:100 instead of 1:200, may be used instead of red-cell pipettes.

2. Discard several drops of the cell suspension, then fill a counting chamber. Place the chamber in a closed Petri dish containing a damp filter paper; let stand 15 minutes to allow the platelets to settle.

3. Platelets are best counted by phase-contrast microscopy, but ordinary light microscopy is perfectly adequate if the count is carefully done. Special care must be taken so that the diluting fluid is not contaminated either with dirt particles or bacteria, both of which may simulate platelets.

4. The number is determined by counting platelets in the 25 small squares of the erythrocyte counting area (1 sq mm) on both sides of the chamber and multiplying the total number counted by 1000. If the Unopette is used, the multiple is 500 when both sides of the chamber are counted.

Electronic Methods

Electronic methods are commonly used to count platelets in platelet-rich plasma and in whole blood. With plasma methods, counts are done on platelet-rich plasma samples and converted mathematically to a whole-blood platelet count. This conversion is based on the patient's hematocrit and a correction factor for platelets trapped by red cells during sedimentation or centrifugation. The major source of difficulty with the plasma methods is in the separation of red cells from the platelet-rich plasma. Increased numbers of red cells in the test plasma result in falsely low platelet counts. With the new Coulter Counter models and the Technician system, platelets are counted in whole blood, which is automatically diluted with a diluent provided with the system. Mean platelet volume is also provided by these instruments.

Electronic methods for counting platelets are much quicker and more reproducible than manual methods. When done carefully, they are probably more accurate for most laboratories, but these methods have not overcome the errors caused by platelet clumping and bizarre platelets. Marked variation in platelet size may affect counts obtained with electronic methods. Some of our experience comparing counts on platelet-rich plasma, using an electronic particle counter, with manual counting, using a phase microscope, is shown in Table 5-1. Correlation is poorest in samples that contain large platelets. This demonstrates the importance of comparing platelet numbers as estimated from the smear with platelet counts.

TABLE 5-1. Comparison of Platelet Counts Performed Manually (phase) and Electronically

Sample	Manual/Phase	Electronic
1	293,000	240,000
2	89,000	84,000
3	248,000	300,000
4	523,000	588,000
5	379,000	391,000
6	293,000	265,000
7	118,000	104,000
8	157,000	134,000
9*	425,000	335,000
10*	325,000	265,000

* Large platelets.

Normal Value: 150,000 to 400,000 Range of error (light microscopy) 16 to 25% Range of error (phase microscopy) 11 to 15% Range of error (electronic) 1.2 to 4%

References

Brecher G, and Cronkite EP: Morphology of human blood platelets. J Appl Physiol 3:365, 1950.
Hardisty RM, and Ingram GIC: Bleeding Disorders. Investigation and Management. Philadelphia, F.A. Davis, 1965, p. 269.
Wertz RK, and Koepke JA: A critical analysis of platelet counting methods. Am J Clin Pathol 68:195, 1977.

MEASUREMENT OF PLATELET ADHESIVENESS

General Principles

The initial step of hemostasis involves adherence of platelets to damaged vessels. Subsequently, platelet aggregates also form at the site of injury. Tests of platelet adhesiveness can be divided into two groups; those measuring adhesion alone, which may involve exposing platelet-rich plasma to glass slides and cover slips, and tests that measure both adhesion and aggregation. Tests measuring adhesion and aggregation are the most practical and include the in vivo method of Borchgrevink and the in vitro methods using glass bead columns.

In Vivo Methods

The adequacy of in vivo adhesiveness can be estimated by comparing the platelet count done on anticoagulated blood with a platelet count done on blood obtained from a superficial cut made on the volar surface of the forearm when doing a bleeding time. A standardized linear cut (10 mm by 1 mm) has been recommended by Borchgrevink for this test. Didisheim and Bunting have modified this procedure by using a 5-mm-deep incision made with a No. 11 Bard-Parker blade. Starting 1 minute after the incision is made and continuing until bleeding stops, serial platelet counts are done at 2-minute intervals. The site is gently wiped with gauze one-half minute before each collection. The results are averaged, and the average count is subtracted from the count performed on the anticoagulated sample to obtain the number of adhesive platelets, which is then expressed as a percentage of the whole.

Normal Values: Borchgrevink's method: 24 to 58% adhesive platelets. Didisheim and Bunting's method: 15 to 45% adhesive platelets. Patients with severe impairment of this platelet function may have only 10% adhesive platelets. Reduced platelet adhesiveness is usually associated with a prolonged bleeding time.

References

Borchgrevink CF: A method for measuring platelet adhesiveness in vivo. Acta Med Scand *168:*157, 1960.
Borchgrevink CF: Platelet adhesion in vivo in patients with bleeding disorders. Acta Med Scand *170:*231, 1961.
Bowie EJW, Thompson JH, Didisheim P, and Owen CA Jr: Mayo Clinic Laboratory Manual of Hemostasis. Philadelphia, W.B. Saunders 1971 pp. 39-47.
Owen CA Jr, Bowie EJW, Didisheim P, and Thompson JH Jr: The Diagnosis of Bleeding Disorders. Boston, Little, Brown & Co., 1969, pp. 80-81.

In Vitro Methods—Glass-Bead Retention

Several methods introduced for the determination of in vitro quantitative platelet adhesiveness depend on the fact that platelets are normally retained or trapped between glass beads when native whole blood, anticoagulated whole blood, or platelet-rich plasma is passed through a column containing small glass beads. This involves both adhesion and aggregation, and results are expressed as the percentage of platelets retained in the columns. The first of these tests to become popular was the Salzman test (1963). This method involved a comparison of venous platelet counts in whole blood collected by Vacutainers directly into EDTA and whole blood added to EDTA after first passing through a glass bead column that contained a specific quantity of glass beads. Results with this method showed decreased retention in patients with von Willebrand's disease, thrombasthenia, and other platelet function defects. Efforts have been made to standardize the test by using a motor-driven device to control the flow rate of the blood through the glass bead columns, since platelet adhesiveness in patients with abnormal platelet function becomes normal if the rate of flow is too slow. Whether or not anticoagulant is used, the flow rate of the blood through the glass bead column, the size and amount of glass beads, plasma cofactors, hematocrit, and the mechanical fragility of red cells have all been shown to influence the results obtained. Because of this, these tests lack specific diagnostic value, but may, when combined with the bleeding time, serve as one of the best tools to substantiate a diagnosis of von Willebrand's disease. In some instances, the platelet-retention test may be the only abnormal finding, since it is not affected by medication, pregnancy, or transfusion. With increasing interest in hypercoagulability, the test has been altered by using glass bead columns with less surface in an effort to demonstrate hyperadhesiveness.

In Vitro Platelet Adhesiveness Test (Method of Salzman) (Retention in Glass Bead Column)

Equipment

1. Superbrite-type 070 Glass Beads.
   Source: 1. Cataphote Corp., Jackson, MS
            2. Potter's Industries, Inc., Carlstad, NJ
2. Tygon tubing (0.025 ID × .031 wall).
3. Nylon-hose (stocking) filter (wash hose in a 10% silicone solution and dry).
4. 1 ML/ML adapter (B-D No. 3113).
5. 2 Vacutainer (B-D) tubes containing EDTA.
6. 2 Vacutainer (B-D) holders.
7. 2 Vacutainer Luer-adapters (B-D No. 5731).
8. 1 20-gauge Luer needle.
9. Alternately, glass bead filters from Diagnostica, Inc. Miami, FL could be used.

Procedure

1. Fill an 11-inch piece of tygon tubing with 2.6 g of glass beads. Seal one end with a piece of nylon and a Luer adapter and the other with nylon and an ML/ML adapter. Alternative columns:
   Adeplat S (for decreased adhesiveness)
                  65 cm$_2$ surface
   Adeplat T (for increased adhesiveness)
                  45 cm$_2$ surface
2. Assemble the equipment before performing the venipuncture (Figure 5-1). An uncomplicated venipuncture and a free flow of blood are essential for a valid test.
3. For the test sample, thread the Luer adapter attached to the tubing securely into the Vacutainer (B-D) holder and place the Vacutainer tube in the holder until the leading edge of the stopper is just even with the line on the holder. The tube will retract slightly. Leave the tube in this position.
4. For the control sample, thread the Luer adapter securely into the second Vacutainer holder, and place the second Vacutainer tube in the holder until the leading edge of the stopper is just even with the line on the holder. The tube will retract slightly. Leave the tube in this position.
5. Cleanse the venipuncture site in the anticubital fossa. Apply a tourniquet.
6. Attach the sterile 20-gauge Luer needle to the ML/ML adapter on the plastic tubing. Perform a venipuncture in the usual manner. Place two

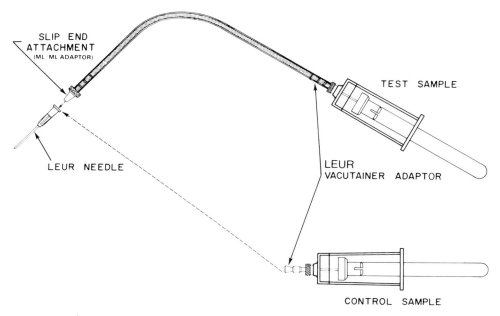

Figure 5-1. Equipment for the in vitro platelet adhesiveness test of Salzman.

fingers behind the flange of the Vacutainer holder and push the Vacutainer tube onto the needle with the thumb of the same hand. Blood will not be visible until the tube is in proper position and the needle is in the lumen of the vein. Gently agitate the Vacutainer tube during blood collection. The tube should fill in 40 to 50 seconds. If more than 1 minute is required, the sample should be discarded, and the test repeated, utilizing another venipuncture at a different site.

7. After cessation of blood flow into the Vacutainer tube, disconnect the glass bead column from the needle in the vein and attach the assembly for the control sample to the Luer needle. Using the Vacutainer technique, collect the control sample.
8. Remove the tourniquet and remove the needle from the vein.
9. Gently invert both samples several times to mix thoroughly with anticoagulant.
10. Perform a platelet count on each blood sample.

Calculation

Platelet Retention (%) =

$$\frac{\text{Initial Platelet Count} - \text{Final Platelet Count}}{\text{Initial Platelet Count}} \times 100$$

Normal Value: To be determined by individual laboratory according to type of columns used. With column made according to description with procedure, retained platelets are >25%.

References

Salzman ER: Measurement of platelet adhesiveness: a simple in vitro technique demonstrating an abnormality in von Willebrand's disease. J Lab Clin Med 62:724, 1963.

Strauss HS, and Bloom GE: von Willebrand's disease. N Engl J Med 273:171, 1965.

Sullivan JM, Heinle RA, and Garlin R: Studies of platelet adherence, glucose tolerance and serum lipoprotein patterns in patients with coronary artery disease. Am J Med Sci 264:475, 1972.

Modification of Salzman's Test (Bowie, et al) (Retention in Glass Bead Column)

Equipment and Reagents

1. Superbrite = type 070 Glass Beads.
   Source: 1. Cataphote Corp., Jackson, MS
   2. Potter's Industries, Inc., Carlstad, NJ
2. Tygon tubing (.025 ID × .031 wall).
3. 2 ML/ML adapters (B.D. No. 3113).
4. Nylon-hose (stocking) filter (wash hose in a 10% silicone solution and dry).
5. Sodium heparin—1000 U/ml.
6. Plastic snap-cap tubes (12 × 75 mm), each containing 0.1 ml of 4% dipotassium EDTA, which has been allowed to dry.
7. Plastic test tube with snap-cap (17 × 100 mm).
8. 2 plastic syringes (20 ml).
9. Infusion pump (for example, model 351 Sage Instruments).
10. Platelet counting facility (phase-contrast microscope or electronic counter).
11. Alternatively, glass bead columns from Diagnostica, Inc., Miami, FL could be used.

Procedure

1. Fill an 11-inch piece of tygon tubing with 2.6 g of glass beads. Seal at each end with a small piece of silicone-coated nylon and the ML/ML adapters. Alternative filters:

   Adeplat S (for decreased adhesiveness)
       65 cm² surface
   Adeplat T (for increased adhesiveness)
       45 cm² surface

2. Draw 12 ml of blood in a plastic syringe by a clean venipuncture. Place 2 ml in a snap-cap EDTA tube for the control platelet-count and place the remainder in a 17 × 100 mm plastic tube that contains 0.04 ml of sodium heparin as anticoagulant (4 U/ml of whole blood). Mix the blood with the anticoagulant by inverting the tube at least 6 times.
   Note: If other hematologic tests are ordered, such as CBC or retics, the initial platelet count may be done from the EDTA Vacutainer tube.
3. Draw 10 ml of the heparinized blood into a plastic (20 ml) syringe. Place the syringe in the infusion pump and attach the glass bead column to the end of the syringe by a ½-inch piece of tygon tubing. Adjust the infusion pump to push the plunger of the syringe so that blood is passed through the glass bead column at a constant rate of 6 ml/min. With Adeplat columns, use 4 ml/min.

4. As the blood exudes from the end of the column, collect the first 3 ml in a test tube and discard. Collect the next 2 ml (4 and 5) in the special tube containing 0.1 ml EDTA (page 209). With Adeplat columns, discard the first 2 ml and collect the third ml in the special tube containing 0.05 ml EDTA instead of 0.1 ml. The EDTA prevents platelet aggregation, which might interfere with subsequent counting.
5. Do platelet counts on these samples and that collected for the initial platelet count.
6. Calculate the percentage of platelets remaining in the column:

Platelet Retention (%) =

$$\frac{\text{Initial Platelet Count} - \text{Final Platelet Count}}{\text{Initial Platelet Count}} \times 100$$

Normal Values: >70% retained platelets with column made as described; 59 to 99% retained platelets with Adeplat S; 3 to 38% retained platelets with Adeplat T.

Technical Hints

1. Heparin should be used as the anticoagulant.
2. If hematocrit value is less than 35%, platelet retention will be low by this technique.
3. A clean venipuncture and a good flow of blood are important.
4. To demonstrate the difference between normal and von Willebrand's disease, it is necessary to standardize the flow rate accurately.

References

Bowie EJW, Owen CA Jr, Thompson JH Jr, and Didisheim P: Platelet adhesiveness in von Willebrand's disease. Am J Clin Pathol 52:69, 1969.
Bowie EJW, Thompson JH Jr, Didisheim P, and Owen CA Jr: Mayo Clinic Laboratory Manual of Hemostasis. Philadelphia, W.B. Saunders, 1971, p. 43.

OBSERVATION OF THE CLOT

Procedure (Figure 5-2)

1. Draw 10 ml of blood in a syringe and place 5 ml in each of 2 graduated glass centrifuge tubes.
2. Insert 2 wooden applicator sticks in each and allow the blood to stand at room temperature for 4 hours.
3. At the end of this time, gently remove the clots that are attached to the applicator sticks. Loosen clots gently if they are stuck to the tubes.
4. Note the number of drops of serum that escape from each clot when it is held in a vertical position. This is referred to as serum "drip-out." The normal clot is relatively dry, and the rate of serum "drip-out" is 2 drops or less in 2 minutes.
5. Observe the volume of serum and red blood cells that have spontaneously escaped from the clots. In a patient with a normal hematocrit value, the clot usually occupies 50 to 60% of the original volume, leaving 40% or

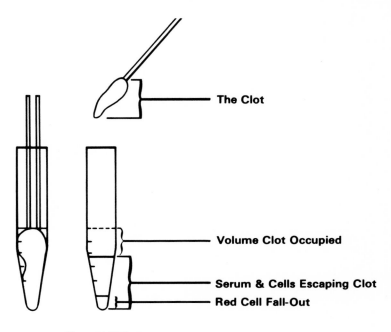

The Clot

Volume Clot Occupied

Serum & Cells Escaping Clot
Red Cell Fall-Out

Normal Values

Drip out---------------------------------- **Less than 2 drops @ 2 mins.**
Volume clot occupied ---------------------- **40 - 60 %**
Serum and cells escaping ------------------ **Over 40 %**
Red cell fall-out ----------------------------**0 - 5 %**
Serum retained in clot ----------------------**Less than 20 %**

Figure 5-2. Observation of the clot. Procedure for removal of the clot, measurement of serum and cells escaping clot, red cell fallout, and serum retained in clot.

        more of serum and cells. Less than 40% volume of serum and cells is abnormal.

6. Notice the red cell fallout. If it is below the 0.1 ml mark, it is negligible. If it is over 0.2 ml, centrifuge the tube and measure the exact volume. Less than 5% (0.25 ml) is normal.

7. A normal clot is firm, tightly attached to the applicator stick, and elastic.

8. If the hematocrit value is known, it is possible to determine the percentage of serum retained in the clot by the following calculation:

(1) Volume of clot (%) =

$$\frac{\text{Total vol blood (ml)} - \text{Vol of serum and RBCs escaping clot (ml)}}{\text{Total volume of blood (ml)}} \times 100$$

(2) Serum retained in clot (%) =
[Vol of clot (%) + RBC fallout (%)] − [Hematocrit (%)]

Normal Values: Amount of serum and red blood cells escaping clot = 40% or more. Red cell fallout = less than 5%. Serum retained in clot = less than 20%. Serum "drip-out" = 2 drops or less in 2 minutes. If there is significant variation between the two tests, report the one that is most nearly normal.

Interpretation (Photographs courtesy of Dr. L.W. Diggs)

The amount of serum expression is decreased in thrombocytopenia and thrombasthenia, even in heterozygotes. In addition, the clot tends to be soft and friable, and there may be increased serum "drip-out" (Figure 5-3). It is well to remember, how-

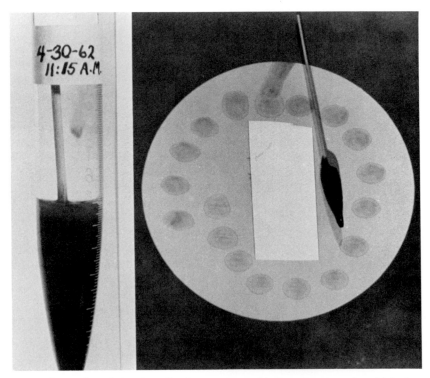

Figure 5-3.   Observation of the clot. Clot from patient with thrombocytopenia, which shows poor retraction and is soft and friable with increased serum "drip-out."

ever, that the size and character of the clot are influenced not only by platelet activity but also by the quantity and reactivity of the fibrinogen and the volume of red blood cells. A small, firm clot with increased red cell fallout suggests hypofibrinogenemia (Figure 5-4). With congenital dysfibrinogenemia (Figure 5-5), red cell fallout is increased, but the clot is of normal size. Red cell fallout is also significantly increased in polycythemia. Fibrinolysis may be suggested by increased red cell fallout, but usually only small strands of clot remain (Figure 5-6). Because of delayed clotting in hemophilia, the clot is layered with a plasma clot at the top and a whole-blood clot at the bottom (Figure 5-7). In cryoglobulinemia, there is no serum expression (Figure 5-8).

Reference

Diggs LW: Observation of the clot. Memphis & Mid-South Med J 37:381, 1962.

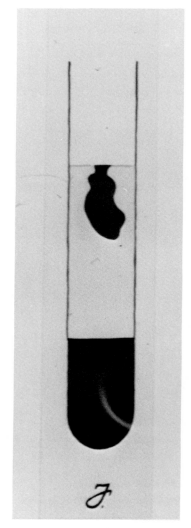

Figure 5-4. Observation of the clot. Diagram of clot from patient with hypofibrinogenemia, which shows a small clot with increased red cell fallout.

PLATELET AGGREGATION

General Principles

Born and Cross found that the optical density of platelet-rich plasma (PRP) less that of platelet-free plasma was proportional to the concentration of platelets. Their turbidimetric method for continuously recording platelet aggregation in PRP is based on this observation. Platelet aggregation depends on agitating platelets in the presence of calcium, fibrinogen, and an aggregating agent as shown in Figure 5-9. When aggregating agents such as arachidonic acid, ADP, epinephrine (Adrenalin, Parke-

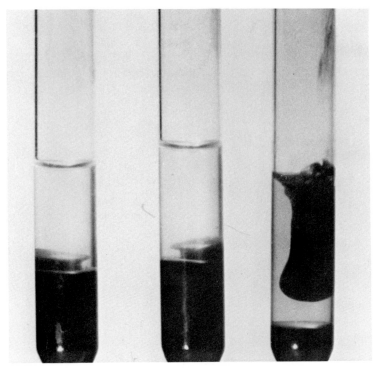

Figure 5-5.   Observation of the clot. Clot from a patient with dysfibrinogenemia, which is of normal size with increased red cell fallout.

Davis), collagen, and ristocetin are added to platelet-rich plasma, normal platelets rapidly form aggregates, which produces a change in the light transmission of the sample. This process can be measured spectrophotometrically and recorded. As more and more aggregates are formed, more light can pass through the solution, producing a progressive deflection of the recorder from the baseline. This deflection represents an increase in light transmission that is proportional to the degree of aggregation.

When PRP is stirred, it swirls because of the discoid shape of the platelets. Swirling of the PRP is macroscopically visible and is responsible for the wide oscillations of the light transmission baseline (Figure 5-10). When an aggregating agent is added, the baseline immediately narrows (Figure 5-10) as the platelets become spherical and the swirling stops. Light transmission increases as platelet clumps form. Coarse oscillation may again be seen when large platelet-clumps pass through the light path near the peak of the light-transmission curve (Figure 5-10).

Arachidonic acid produces primary aggregation and is useful as a screening aggregating agent because it requires the normal activity of the cyclo-oxygenase enzyme in platelets to be converted to thromboxane A_2, which is a potent platelet aggregator. Aspirin is a strong inhibitor of cyclo-oxygenase, so the absence of arachidonic acid aggregation gives good evidence of such a drug effect. When

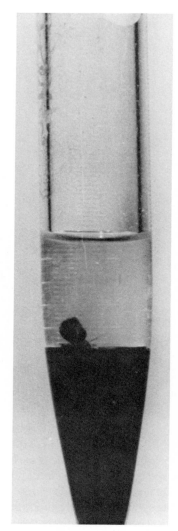

Figure 5-6. Observation of the clot. Clot from a patient with increased fibrinolysis, which shows almost complete liquefaction of the clot with only a few small strands of intact clot remaining.

arachidonic acid aggregation is absent, it is usually unnecessary to continue aggregation tests until the drug status of the patient has been determined.

ADP-induced aggregation may occur in either one or two phases or the first and second phases may be fused. Large second phases are usually irreversible. Figure 5-10 shows rapid disaggregation of aggregates induced by low-concentration ADP (1.07 μg/ml) with only a small second phase seen on the downslope of the tracing. Such rapid disaggregation (>50% at 3 minutes after maximum light transmission occurred) was found in the laboratory of Dr. James Davis in the PRP of 45% of 150 men with no known occlusive vascular disease. Only 20% of 95 men with occlusive

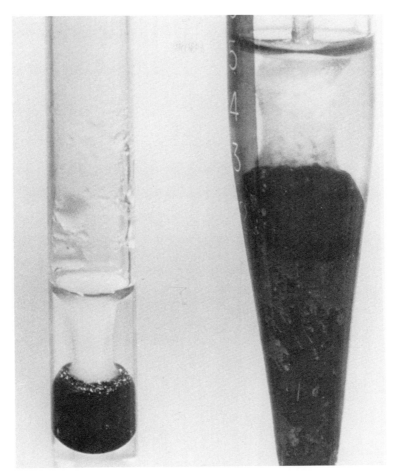

Figure 5-7. Observation of the clot. Clot from a patient with hemophilia, which shows a layer of clotted plasma over a whole blood clot.

vascular diseases had such rapid disaggregation. None of these 245 men gave a history of a bleeding tendency or of use of aspirin within the week preceding their tests. Although rapid disaggregation has been reported to be associated with some hemorrhagic diseases, including von Willebrand's disease, its frequent occurrence in the PRP of normal men makes rapid disaggregation of doubtful significance in the pathogenesis of hemorrhagic states.

Epinephrine (Adrenalin, Parke-Davis) induced platelet aggregation may normally occur in either one or two phases and is largely irreversible. With the final concentration of Epinephrine (Adrenalin) (5 μg/ml), a second phase is usually induced in normal PRP. Figure 5-11 illustrates blocking of a large second phase of Adrenalin-induced platelet aggregation by aspirin. The first phase is essentially unchanged after aspirin ingestion. Adrenalin-induced aggregation is sometimes absent in patients

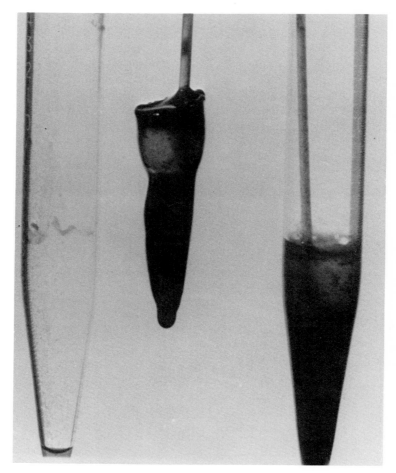

Figure 5-8.   Observation of the clot. Clot from a patient with cryoglobulinemia, which shows the solidification of the plasma with no serum expression.

who appear to be totally normal and may be related to the temporary saturation of catecholamine binding sites on platelets.

When a suspension of collagen is added to stirred PRP (Figure 5-12), there is a lag period before aggregation occurs in a single, irreversible phase (upper tracing of Figure 5-12). Aspirin ingestion inhibits the platelet release reaction and may strikingly inhibit, but not abolish, the aggregation produced by the collagen suspension (lower tracing of Figure 5-12). A biphasic response to collagen after aspirin ingestion has been observed in a few instances (lower tracing of Figure 5-12).

When ristocetin is added to PRP, aggregation normally occurs rapidly, with no distinct primary and secondary phases present. Coarse oscillations are seen because of the large platelet clumps that are formed.

The relationships of the in vitro platelet-aggregation tests to in vivo platelet function are not clear. Since the hemostatic platelet plug formed in response to injury of a

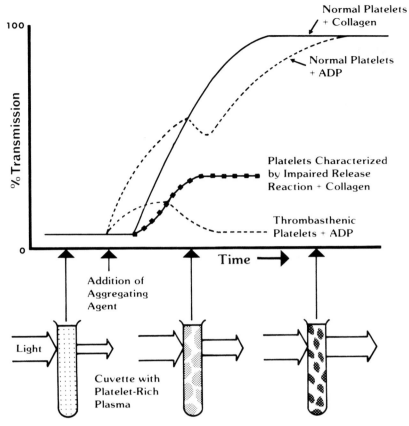

Figure 5-9.   Platelet aggregation.

blood vessel appears to depend on adherence of platelets to exposed connective tissue and the release of ADP and other substances from the adherent platelets, leading to aggregation of other platelets, collagen-induced platelet aggregation in PRP may be the best in vitro indicator of platelet hemostatic activity.

Technique

Equipment

Platelet aggregometer with a recorder. (We use a Chrono-log aggregometer and recorder; Chrono-log Corp., Havertown, PA.)

Reagents

1. Sodium citrate solution—3.8% (silicone-coated Vacutainer (B-D) tubes containing 3.8% sodium citrate may be used).
2. Arachidonic acid (Bio/Data Corp., Horsham, PA). Reconstitute vial with 0.5 ml distilled water (working concentration 5 mg/ml). Stable for 24

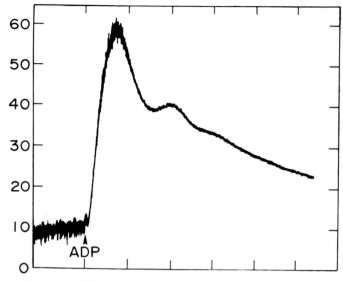

Figure 5-10. Tracing made during aggregation of platelets in platelet-rich plasma with ADP.

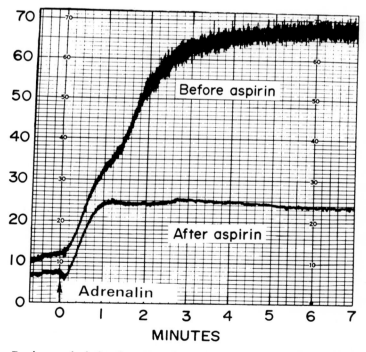

Figure 5-11. Tracings made during the aggregation of platelets with adrenalin in platelet-rich plasma from a patient tested before and after the administration of aspirin.

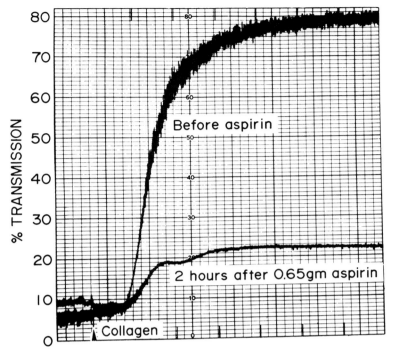

Figure 5-12. Tracings made during aggregation of platelets with collagen in platelet-rich plasma from a patient tested before and after the administration of aspirin.

hours at 2 to 8°C and longer at −20°C. Vial must be kept stoppered at all times. (Final concentration in test system approximately 0.5 mg/ml.)

3.   ADP—adenosine-5′-diphosphate, disodium salt (Sigma Chem. Co., St. Louis, MO). STOCK—Dissolve 11.8 mg in 10 ml of barbital buffer. Store frozen in 0.5 ml aliquots and thaw just before use. Prepare "strong" working solution by diluting STOCK ADP 1 : 10 with normal saline (final concentration in test system 10.7 μg/ml). Prepare "weak" solution by diluting the "strong" solution 1 : 10 with normal saline (final concentration in the test system 1.07 μg/ml).

4.   Adrenalin chloride solution (Parke-Davis, Detroit, MI) 1 mg/ml. Dilute 0.1 ml to 1.82 ml with normal saline. Prepare just before use and discard when test is completed. (Final concentration in test system 5.0 μg/ml.)

5.   Modified Tyrode's solution (contains no calcium or magnesium). A solution containing 8 g NaCl, 0.2 gm KCl, 1 g NaHCO$_3$, 0.05 g NaH$_2$PO$_4$•H$_2$O and 1 g glucose is prepared with deionized water. After the pH is adjusted to 7.35 with 0.1 N HCl, the volume is brought to 1 L.

6.   Collagen (Sigma Chem. Co., St. Louis, MO). A suspension of 2 g of collagen in 100 ml of modified Tyrode's solution is blended in a regular blender for 10 periods of 30 seconds each, with 5 minutes between each blending period to avoid overheating. After blending, the mixture is centrifuged for

5 minutes at 2000 rpm to remove large particles. The supernatant suspension is diluted with modified Tyrode's solution and tested with normal PRP until the minimum concentration that produces maximum aggregation has been found (usually, in the range of 1 part suspension to 9 parts of modified Tyrode's solution). The undiluted suspension is kept refrigerated at approximately 5°C until needed. (Further dilution to 1:20 and 1:40 may be used for hypercoagulability studies.)

7. Ristocetin (Helena Laboratories, Beaumont, TX). Reconstitute vial with distilled water (working concentration 15 mg/ml). Allow to stand 5 minutes at room temperature for complete dissolution. Stable for 4 hours at room temperature or for 1 month at −20°C. (Final concentration in test system approximately 1.5 mg/ml.) For study of patients with variant von Willebrand's (type IIB), use a final concentration of approximately 0.5 mg/ml. A final concentration of 1.0 mg/ml is considered by some to be more useful in the detection of patients with mild von Willebrand's disease.

Preparation of Blood Samples

1. Using the Vacutainer (B-D) system, draw about 2 ml blood into a red-stoppered Vacutainer tube. Remove this tube from the adapter and discard. Insert siliconized Vacutainer tubes containing sodium citrate and allow to fill to 5 ml. Alternatively, using the two-syringe technique, draw blood into a plastic syringe and place 4.5 ml in a plastic test tube containing 0.5 ml of 3.8% solution of sodium citrate.

2. Centrifuge blood sample for 10 minutes at 1000 rpm at room temperature to obtain platelet-rich plasma (PRP) (10 minutes at minimum speed, "0" setting, on Clay Adams' Dynac centrifuge).

3. Carefully remove tube from centrifuge. Using a plastic pipette system, withdraw with care as much plasma as possible. This is PRP. Keep plasma in a plastic tube at room temperature and test within 3 hours after phlebotomy.

4. To obtain platelet-poor plasma (PPP), re-spin blood sample at room temperature for 10 minutes at 3000 rpm (10 minutes at maximum setting on Clay Adams' Dynac centrifuge). Using a plastic pipette system, withdraw with care as much of the plasma as possible.

Procedure (For use with Chrono-log aggregometer and recorder)

1. Prepare aggregating agents to be used in testing.

2. To an aggregometer cuvette add 0.4 ml of PPP. Insert into aggregometer and adjust baseline of recorder to "10." This recording provides a baseline for maximum aggregation. (The direction of recording can be changed by reversing the leads connecting the recorder to the aggregometer.)

3. Remove the cuvette and replace it with one in which 0.4 ml PRP and a magnetic stirrer are added. Adjust baseline of recorder to "90." Allow the baseline to record for about 1 minute.

4. Add 0.04 ml of one of the aggregating agents prepared as has been described and continue to record at least until after light transmission no longer increases; or in the case of "weak" ADP, record disaggregation as the downslope of the light transmission curve that usually follows aggregation.

Precautions

1. Test should be done on specimens from fasting patients.
2. A clean venipuncture, free of hemolysis is essential.
3. Blood samples and plasma should be kept at room temperature and tested within 3 hours.
4. Plastic tubes or siliconized glassware must be used throughout the entire plasma preparation process. We use siliconized Vacutainers (B-D No. A3204SW).
5. Normal ranges should be established in each laboratory with the reagents used. More than one strength of ADP may be useful, and varying dilutions of collagen are particularly useful in detecting hypercoagulability. Collagen varies with the type and age of the product used. Available preparations of arachidonic acid, ADP, epinephrine (Adrenalin, Parke-Davis), and ristocetin are more consistent.
6. Arachidonic acid aggregation should be performed first. Normal response time is 15 to 30 seconds. If there is no aggregation, further testing need not be done until the drug status of the patient has been determined.
7. When indicated, ristocetin aggregation should be performed as soon as possible because the agglutination reaction that occurs upon addition of ristocetin to platelets is dependent on the pH of the plasma, which changes as the plasma remains at room temperature.
8. Epinephrine (Adrenalin) aggregation should be the last performed, for studies show that the response to this agent seems to increase after the platelet-rich plasma has been sitting at room temperature for 60 minutes.
9. Always use at least two different aggregating agents, preferably arachidonic acid and collagen, except when testing for von Willebrand's conditions when ristocetin should also be included.
10. The best way to detect drug effect, such as that due to aspirin, is to use arachidonic acid. With the use of epinephrine (Adrenalin, Parke-Davis) as an aggregating agent, the second phase will be absent with aspirin ingestion. These changes are particularly important in evaluating ristocetin aggregation, which is also affected to some degree by aspirin. When abnormal responses occur with more than one aggregating agent, it is helpful to include aggregation with ristocetin.

Interpretation

The response to platelet aggregation can be expressed quantitatively, in terms of maximum change in light transmission and rate of change or "slope," or descriptively. Factors that affect the response are the way in which samples are drawn and processed, the concentrations and activity of the reagents, as well as abnormalities in platelets themselves. For each instrument system and reagent, a range of optimum responses must be determined. As shown in Figure 5-13, reports can include the following:

Platelet Aggregation

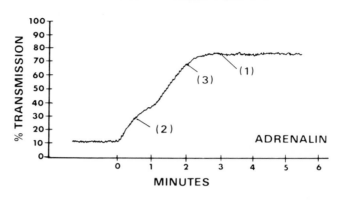

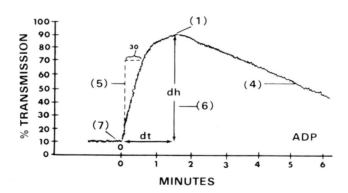

(1) **Maximum aggregation**, (2) **Primary phase**,
(3) **Second phase**, (4) **Disaggregation**,
(5) **Slope**, (6) **Aggregation Index, AI** $= \frac{dh}{dt}$
(7) **Addition of aggregating agent**.

Figure 5-13. Ways of reporting platelet aggregation.

1. Percent of Maximum Aggregation. This is the degree of change in light transmission produced by the addition of an aggregating reagent when compared to the percent of transmission of platelet-poor plasma (PPP), which is considered to be 100% aggregation, and that through platelet-rich plasma (PRP), which is considered to be 0% aggregation.

2. Primary Phase.   This is the initial response to an aggregating agent.

3. Second Phase.   This is visible additional aggregation in response to the release of endogenous ADP; normally seen with aggregation induced by epinephrine (Adrenalin, B-D) and low concentrations of ADP, but not with arachidonic acid, collagen, and ristocetin (seen in von Willebrand's disease with ristocetin).

4. Percent of Disaggregation.   This is the percentage of fall from maximum aggregation in a 10-minute period after initiation of aggregation.

5. Slope.   This is the rise in millimeters over a 30-second period on the steepest portion of the curve.

6. Aggregation Index.   This is the distance in millimeters from the peak of maximum aggregation to the baseline (dh) divided by the length in millimeters of a line extending from the point of the addition of the aggregating agent to its interception with dh (dt):

$$AI = \frac{dh}{dt}$$

Primary phase aggregation with arachidonic acid, ADP, epinephrine (Adrenalin, Parke-Davis), and collagen is absent in patients with homozygous thrombasthenia, and heterozygotes for this condition may show a diminished response. A single dose of aspirin results in the complete absence of arachidonic acid aggregation for as long as 5 days and a delayed response time up to 8 days. Platelets from patients with storage-pool disease may aggregate normally or abnormally with arachidonic acid.

Variable abnormalities in second-phase aggregation are seen in inherited disorders such as storage-pool disease and "aspirin-like" defects and in patients who have taken aspirin or related drugs. The degree of abnormality depends on the specific condition and, in the case of drug effects, the time of ingestion of the drugs. Second-phase aggregation with epinephrine (Adrenalin, Parke-Davis) may be completely inhibited if as little as one aspirin tablet is ingested on the day the testing is done, but variable inhibition is found when testing is done at intervals after ingestion. Failure of platelets to aggregate in response to epinephrine (Adrenalin, Parke-Davis) may occur in the PRP of some patients with polycythemia vera or thrombocytosis and also in patients who have no obvious disease state. It may be seen in persons under stress and in those taking adrenergic drugs.

Ristocetin aggregation is particularly useful in the diagnosis of patients who have von Willebrand's disease and the Bernard-Soulier syndrome. In most such patients, aggregation is normal with arachidonic acid, ADP, epinephrine (Adrenalin, Parke-Davis), and collagen, but diminished with ristocetin. The calculation of the aggregation index (AI) for ristocetin aggregation is a valuable addition. It is usually <1.7 in von Willebrand's disease. Ristocetin aggregation of formalized platelets in the presence of test plasma forms the basis of the factor VIIIR:WF Assay (page 145).

Spontaneous or increased aggregation responses may occur in a number of conditions, such as smoking, stress, atherosclerosis, thromboembolism, diabetes, and hypertension. The range of values is so variable, even in the normal population, that the usual aggregation tests appear to be unsuitable for discriminating between normal and abnormal individuals. By using decreasing concentrations of an agent such as collagen, however, it is possible to identify individuals who show responses outside the range seen in normal persons. Table 5-2 gives a summary of studies done in our laboratory on a group of normal individuals who all had good responses to a 1 to 4 dilution of the collagen preparation that we were using routinely at the time these studies were done. With further dilution, increasing percentages of those studied showed a decrease of more than 15% in aggregation magnitude. Such data suggest that the absence of decreasing aggregation with higher dilutions of collagen is suggestive of hyperreactivity of platelets.

TABLE 5-2. Platelet Aggregation With Variable Dilutions of Collagen (normal subjects)

Aggregating Agent		Collagen			
Dilutions		1:4	1:10	1:12	1:16
% Aggregation Magnitude	Range	76-94	52-86	37-83	16-78
	Mean	84	80	75	63
% Subjects showing a decrease of > 15%			20%	33%	55%

References

Born GVR, and Cross MJ: The aggregation of platelets. J Physiol (Lond) *168*:178, 1963.
Brody JI, Levison SP, and Jung CJ: Sickle cell trait and hematuria associated with von Willebrand's syndromes. Ann Intern Med *86*:529, 1977 (Aggregation Index).
Roper P, et al: Effects of time, platelet concentration and sex in human platelet aggregation response. Am J Clin Pathol *71*:263, 1979.
Sirridge MS, et al: Effects of antiplatelet drugs on platelet function tests. Mo Med *96*:212, 1979.
Stuart RK: Platelet function studies in human beings receiving 300 mg of aspirin per day. J Lab Clin Med *75*:463, 1970 (Slope).
Triplett PA, et al: Platelet Function—Laboratory Evaluation and Clinical Application. Chicago, ASCP, 1978.

PLATELET-FACTOR-3 (PF$_3$) AVAILABILITY TESTS

General Principles

The action of platelets is important in blood coagulation. Platelets are the source of platelet factor 3 (PF$_3$), a lipoprotein that is necessary for the efficient activation of factors X and II. In normal intact circulating platelets, the lipoprotein is not available for the coagulation reaction but becomes so when platelets are altered or activated by some stimulus. Such action can be initiated by mechanical fragmentation, which liberates most of the lipid content, or by the addition of a variety of substances, including kaolin and epinephrine (Adrenalin, Parke-Davis). Results indicate that 20 to 25% of the maximal PF$_3$ activity is made available by kaolin activation; this is probably equivalent to the physiologic amount made available during normal clotting.

It is possible to measure PF_3 activity directly by a two-stage technique in which PF_3 is made available by adding kaolin to the patient's platelet-rich plasma and tested for at intervals by adding aliquots of this mixture with calcium to kaolin-activated platelet-poor plasma.

A direct measurement of PF_3 activity can also be made in a one-stage procedure by providing a standard platelet stimulus in the form of kaolin and epinephrine (Adrenalin, Parke-Davis) to a plasma mixture containing a known concentration of the platelets to be tested and having normal coagulation-factor activity. The recalcification time of such a mixture will depend on the availability of PF_3.

The prothrombin consumption test is an indirect test of intrinsic pathway activity and depends on the measurement of the procoagulant activity that remains in serum after coagulation has taken place. This activity is thought to be caused primarily by residual prothrombin. When PF_3 activity is deficient or abnormalities exist in the coagulation factors whose activation results in the conversion of prothrombin to thrombin, the amount of "prothrombin" remaining in serum should be demonstrably increased. The procedure has been used in the United States over 30 years and a wide variety of techniques have been described. The major variations are indicated in Table 5-3. Although there is some question as to exactly what is being measured in

TABLE 5-3.	Variations in Prothrombin Consumption Techniques	
Treatment of Materials	Method	Variable
Quantity of blood in the clotting tubes		1ml or 2 ml
Time of separation of serum from clot after clotting		15 min, 50 min, 1 hr, 2 hr
Incubation of serum after separation		0 to 45 min
Addition of citrate to serum		May or may not
Addition of platelet substitute		May or may not
	Prothrombin time technique	One-stage or two-stage method for determining
	Method of reporting	Seconds % Utilization % Prothrombin
	Fibrinogen source	Purified bovine fibrinogen Adsorbed human plasma Adsorbed rabbit plasma Simplastin A

this one-stage serum prothrombin time (prothrombin or altered products of coagulation) it still appears that the test can be useful in the laboratory diagnosis of patients with bleeding abnormalities, particularly those who have prolonged bleeding times and possible platelet functional disorders. A modification that includes the addition of a platelet substitute to one of the clotting tubes improves the usefulness of the test in detecting defects in platelet function. The test is no longer indicated in the study of patients with possible coagulation-factor defects because of the availability of many superior methods.

Two-Stage Direct Method for PF₃ Availability

Equipment and Reagents

1. Two silicone-coated Vacutainer tubes containing 3.8% sodium citrate.
2. Barbital-buffered saline.
3. Kaolin-50 (suspension of 50 mg kaolin/ml barbital-buffered saline).
4. Kaolin-10 (suspension of 10 mg kaolin/ml barbital-buffered saline).
5. Calcium chloride (0.025M).
6. Two stopwatches.

Preparation of Blood Samples

1. Using the Vacutainer system, draw about 2 ml blood into a red-stoppered Vacutainer tube. Remove this tube from the adapter and discard. Insert Vacutainer tubes containing sodium citrate and allow to fill to 5 ml. If silicone-coated Vacutainer tubes containing citrate are not available, draw blood with a plastic syringe using the two-syringe technique. Place 4.5 ml of blood in siliconized or plastic tubes containing 0.5 ml of a 3.8% sodium citrate solution.
2. Centrifuge tubes for 10 minutes at 1000 rpm. Remove at least 1 ml platelet-rich plasma (PRP) and keep in a stoppered plastic test tube at room temperature.
3. Centrifuge the remaining blood for 10 minutes at 3000 rpm. Remove plasma and place in a plastic tube. This is the platelet-poor plasma (PPP) and can be used for other clotting tests.

Procedure (Figure 5-14)

1. Place a tube containing 3 ml calcium chloride in the 37°C water bath.
2. Place 0.3 ml PPP in each of 2 glass test tubes and prepare the initial substrate mixture by adding 0.1 ml kaolin-10 to one of the tubes.
3. Prepare the generation mixture in a plastic test tube by adding 0.1 ml kaolin-50 to 1.0 ml PRP.
4. Start a stopwatch and place the generation mixture and initial substrate mixture in the water bath to incubate. This is considered "0" time.
5. At 4 minutes, add 0.1 ml generation mixture to the "0" time substrate mixture and recalcify immediately with 0.4 ml calcium chloride. Start a second stopwatch. Observe for gel formation and record the clotting time.
6. At 17 minutes, prepare the second substrate mixture (0.1 ml kaolin-10 plus 0.3 ml PPP). Start incubation at 18 minutes and test at 22 minutes, as in step 5.

Normal Values: There should be a decrease of at least 20 seconds from the clotting time of the 4-minute sample to that of the 22-minute sample.

Reference

Hardisty RM, and Hutton RA: The Kaolin clotting time of platelet-rich plasma: A test of platelet factor 3 availability. Br J Haematol 11:258, 1965.

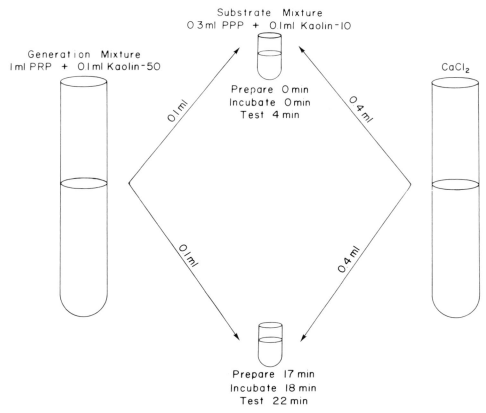

Substrate Mixture
0.3 ml PPP + 0.1 ml Kaolin-10

Generation Mixture
1 ml PRP + 0.1 ml Kaolin-50

CaCl$_2$

Prepare 0 min
Incubate 0 min
Test 4 min

0.1 ml

0.4 ml

0.1 ml

0.4 ml

Prepare 17 min
Incubate 18 min
Test 22 min

Figure 5-14. The two-stage direct method for PF$_3$ availability. A generation mixture containing platelet-rich plasma and a kaolin suspension is incubated for 22 minutes. The release of PF$_3$ is determined by testing aliquots of this mixture after 4 and 22 minutes of incubation. Testing is done by adding 0.1 ml generation mixture and 0.4 ml calcium chloride to substrate mixtures of platelet-poor plasma and kaolin that have each been incubated for 4 minutes.

One-Stage Direct Method for PF$_3$ Availability

Equipment and Reagents

1. Two silicone-coated Vacutainer tubes containing 3.8% sodium citrate.
2. Kaolin (1.5 gm/100 ml barbital-buffered saline).
3. Adrenalin, Parke-Davis (vial of 1.0 ml 1:1000 dilution).
4. Calcium chloride (0.25M).
5. Fibrometer (stopwatch if tilt-tube method is used).

Preparation of Blood Samples

1. Using the vacuum tube system, draw about two ml of blood in red-stoppered Vacutainer tube. Remove this tube from the adapter and discard. Insert Vacutainer tubes containing sodium citrate and allow to fill to 5 ml. If silicone-coated Vacutainer tubes containing citrate are not available, draw blood with a plastic syringe, using the two-syringe technique.

Place 4.5 ml of blood in each of 2 siliconized or plastic test tubes containing 0.5 ml of a 3.8% sodium citrate solution.

2. Centrifuge both tubes for 10 minutes at 1000 rpm. Remove at least 1 ml platelet-rich plasma (PRP) from each tube and keep in plastic tubes at room temperature. This PRP can also be used for aggregation testing.

3. Centrifuge the remaining blood for 10 minutes more at 3000 rpm. Remove plasma and place in a plastic tube. This is the platelet-poor plasma (PPP) and can be used for other clotting tests.

Note: Care must be exercised in obtaining the blood sample. Although intact red cells have no effect on the kaolin clotting time, lysed red cells release phospholipid and will act as liberated platelet factor 3. If this happens, there is some doubt as to the reliability of a normal result.

Procedure

1. Place a tube containing calcium chloride in the 37°C water bath.
2. Do a platelet count on PRP.
3. Dilute PRP to a count of 50,000 with PPP.
4. Place 0.1 ml of the plasma with the 50,000-platelet count into a plastic tube or fibrocup. Add 0.1 ml kaolin and 10 μl Adrenalin to the sample.
5. Incubate for *exactly* 10 minutes.
6. Add 0.1 ml prewarmed CaCl$_2$ and start timer.
7. Average two results for each sample.

Normal Value: 32.4 to 58.4 seconds (mean 43.3).

Reference

Sirridge MS, et al: Effects of antiplatelet drugs on platelet function tests. Mo Med 96:212, 1979.

Prothrombin Consumption Test

Reagents

1. Simplastin A (General Diagnostics, Morris Plains, NJ).
2. Partial thromboplastin reagent.
3. Barbital-buffered saline.

Preparation of Reference Curve

1. Normal Plasma Pool. Using the two-syringe technique (Vacutainers or syringe), draw blood from at least 5 normal individuals and place in tubes containing 3.8% sodium citrate solution. Mix and centrifuge the samples immediately for 10 minutes at 3000 rpm. Remove plasmas and pool. This is the reference plasma for preparation of the prothrombin activity curve.

2. Prepare the reference curve by diluting the pooled normal plasma to concentrations of 50%, 40%, 30%, 20%, 10%, and 5% in barbital-buffered saline as shown in Table 5-4. The undiluted plasma represents 100%.

3. Prewarm Simplastin A at 37°C (minimum of 5 minutes and a maximum of 60 minutes).

TABLE 5-4. Dilution of Plasma Pool for Preparation of the
Reference Curve (Prothrombin) Consumption Test)

Percent concentration	100	50	40	30	20	10	5
Pooled normal plasma (ml)	0.4	0.2	0.4	0.3	0.2	0.1	0.5
Barbital-buffered saline (ml)	0	0.2	0.6	0.7	0.8	0.9	0.95

4. Prewarm plasma or plasma dilutions at 37°C (minimum of 5 minutes and a maximum of 10 minutes).
5. Pipette 0.2 ml of the prewarmed Simplastin A into a test tube.
6. Add 0.1 ml of the pooled normal plasma and start timer. The formation of a clot is the end point. Repeat the test with a second tube of Simplastin A. A fibrometer may be used.
7. Determine the prothrombin time in duplicate for each of the dilutions.
8. Calculate the average clotting time for each dilution.
9. Using linear graph paper, plot the percentage of concentrations on the horizontal axis and the clotting times in seconds on the vertical axis.
10. Draw the best fitting curve (line) through these points.

Procedure

1. Draw 10 ml blood by the two-syringe technique and place 1 ml in each of 3 dry glass test tubes and 4.5 ml in a tube containing 0.5 ml 3.8% sodium citrate solution.
2. Immediately place the 3 tubes containing 1 ml blood into a 37°C water bath. After 2 minutes, add 0.1 ml partial thromboplastin reagent to the third tube and mix well by tipping.
3. Tilt the tubes as in the whole-blood clotting time.
4. Allow the tubes to remain in the water bath for 1 hour after clotting.
5. Centrifuge the tube containing the citrated blood.
6. Remove the plasma and place it in a test tube.
7. Store at 4°C until serum samples are ready for testing.
8. When the serum tubes have incubated for 1 hour, rim the clots and centrifuge all 3 tubes for 5 minutes at 3000 rpm.
9. Remove and pool the serum from tubes 1 and 2 in a glass test tube. Transfer the serum from tube 3 to a second tube.
10. Allow the test plasma and the 2 tubes of serum to incubate at 37°C for 10 minutes.
11. Pipette into each of 6 other glass test tubes 0.2 ml Simplastin A. Place these tubes in the water bath for at least 2 minutes to warm. A fibrometer may be used.
12. Draw up 0.1 ml plasma into a pipette and add it quickly to a tube contain-

ing 0.2 ml Simplastin A and start the timer. The formation of a clot is the end point.

13.   Repeat the test with a second tube of Simplastin A.
14.   Do duplicate determinations on the serum from the first and second serum tubes.
15.   Using the prothrombin activity curve, as prepared above, determine the percentage of prothrombin activity in the test plasma. If the clotting time is shorter than the 100% pool-plasma value, dilute the test plasma 1:2 with barbital-buffered saline, repeat the prothrombin time and multiply the percentage value obtained by the dilution factor.
16.   Using the prothrombin activity curve, determine the percentage of procoagulant activity remaining in the serum sample.
17.   Percentage of consumption is calculated by dividing the percent consumed (percent in test plasma − percent in serum sample) by the percent in the plasma.

$$\% \text{ Consumption} = \frac{\% \text{ Plasma} - \% \text{ Serum}}{\% \text{ Plasma}} \times 100$$

Normal Values: Serum prothrombin time (from tubes 1 and 2) >20 seconds; Serum prothrombin time from tube 3 >45 seconds; Percent consumed >90%.

Interpretation

If prothrombin consumption in tubes 1 and 2 is abnormal, with correction in tube 3 to which partial thromboplastin reagent, which is a platelet substitute, is added, this suggests that decreased PF_3 availability is responsible for the abnormality.

Example

	Tubes 1 & 2	Tube 3
Normal Range	26-37 sec	44-180 sec
Hemophilia A	17 sec	21 sec
Platelet Function Abnormality	11 sec	90 sec

References

Merskey B: The consumption of prothrombin during coagulation. J Clin Pathol 3:130, 1950.
Owen CA Jr, and Thompson JH Jr: Soybean phosphatides in prothrombin-consumption and thromboplastin-generation tests: their use in recognizing "thrombasthenic hemophilia." Am J Clin Pathol 33:197, 1960.
Sussmen LN, Cohen B, and Gettler R: Clinical application of simplified serum prothrombin consumption test. JAMA 156:702, 1954.

CIRCULATING PLATELET AGGREGATES
(Platelet-Count Ratio Method)

General Principles

This method is based on a determination of the ratio of a platelet count performed on platelet-rich plasma from blood collected in a buffered solution of formaldehyde and EDTA to that of platelet-rich plasma from blood collected in buffered EDTA. It is theorized that platelet aggregates present in vivo or formed during the drawing of the sample will be fixed by the formaldehyde and, because of their size, will be spun down with the RBCs during centrifugation. The ratio could not normally exceed 1.0, and normal values were found to be from 0.8 to 1.0. Values lower than this would suggest an enhanced tendency of platelets to clump either in vivo or during the drawing of the sample.

Technique

Reagents

1. 4% formalin. Add 10 ml of 37.2% formaldehyde solution to 90 ml of distilled water.
2. 0.077 M EDTA. Add 28.66 g of disodium ethylenediamine-tetraacetate ($Na_2 C_{10} O_8 N_2 \cdot 2H_2O$) to 750 ml distilled water. Adjust pH to 7.4 and dilute to 1000 ml with distilled water.
3. Concentrated phosphate-buffered saline (PBS). To 1 L of distilled water add 2 g KCl, 2 g KH_2PO_4, 80 g NaCl and 17.3 g $Na_2HPO_4 \cdot 7H_2O$.
4. Buffered EDTA solution. Add 3 ml of 0.77 M EDTA and 5 ml concentrated PBS to 12 ml distilled water. pH = 7.26.
5. Buffered EDTA-formalin solution. Add 3 ml of 0.077 M EDTA, 5 ml of 4% formalin and 2 ml of concentrated PBS to 10 ml of distilled water. pH = 7.36.

Procedure

1. Place 2 ml of buffered EDTA solution in a 3 ml plastic syringe (A) and 2 ml of buffered EDTA-formalin solution in a second 3 ml plastic syringe (B).
2. Using a 21-gauge Venocut TM infusion set (butterfly), draw 0.5 ml blood into the first syringe (A), allowing 2 to 3 drops to escape before attaching the syringe. Remove the syringe and introduce 0.5 ml air into the syringe and invert it 5 times within 30 seconds to mix.
3. Draw a second sample into syringe B and handle it in the same way.
4. Discard 0.1 ml from each syringe and place the remainder in 2 labeled plastic test tubes. Incubate these at room temperature for 15 minutes.
5. Centrifuge both tubes for 10 minutes at 1000 rpm to obtain platelet-rich plasma.
6. Dilute the platelet-rich plasma 1 : 200 in ammonium oxalate and perform platelet counts by phase-contrast microscopy or do platelet counts using a model B or model ZB Coulter Counter.
7. Express results as:

$$\text{Aggregate ratio} = \frac{\text{Platelet count (EDTA-formalin PRP)}}{\text{Platelet count (EDTA PRP)}}$$

Normal Value: 0.8 to 1.

Note: A recent study showed a decrease in the aggregate ratio after cigarette smoking which was prevented by the ingestion of aspirin, so a normal test result may not be valid if the subject has taken aspirin.

References

Davis JW, and Davis RF: Prevention of cigarette smoking-induced platelet aggregate formation by aspirin. Arch Intern Med *141*:206, 1981.

Wu KK: Platelet hyperaggregability and thrombosis in patients with thrombocythemia. Ann Intern Med *88*:7, 1978.

Wu KK, and Hoak JC: A new method for the quantitative detection of platelet aggregates in patients with arterial insufficiency. Lancet 2:924, 1974.

MEASUREMENT OF PLATELET FACTOR 4 (PF$_4$) AND β-THROMBOGLOBULIN (B-TG) IN PLASMA

General Principles

Platelet factor 4 (PF$_4$) and β-thromboglobulin (B-TG) are platelet-specific proteins secreted from the alpha granules into the circulation when platelets undergo the release reaction. Increased plasma levels of these proteins suggest platelet activation in vivo and may occur in a variety of disorders, including myocardial infarction and coronary artery disease. The presence of these proteins in plasma can be determined by use of competitive binding radioimmunoassay procedures.

Technique for Measurement of PF$_4$

Equipment

1. Thrombotect tube (Abbott #7203). This is an evacuated tube containing EDTA, 2-chloradenosine, and procaine hydrochlorate.
2. Gamma scintillation counter.
3. Centrifuge capable of 2500 × g (centrifuge must be refrigerated if thrombotect tubes are not used to collect specimens).
4. Crushed ice and water bath.
5. Precision pipettes with disposable tips (50, 250, and 500 μl capacity).
6. Plastic test tubes (12 × 75 mm).
7. Vortex mixer.

Reagents (Reagents are included in PF$_4$/RIA kit from Abbott Laboratories)

1. I-125 platelet factor 4 in dilution buffer with stabilizer (contains 0.35 μCi or less/ml).
2. Platelet-factor-4 antiserum (goat) in dilution buffer.
3. Platelet-factor-4 (human) standards: 10, 30, 50, and 100 ng/ml in dilution buffer.
4. Dilution buffer—0.01 M Tris buffer with 0.15 M sodium chloride, containing bovine serum albumin. Preservative: 0.02% sodium azide.
5. Ammonium sulfate (74% saturated) in distilled water.

Collection and Preparation of Samples

1. Prepare a mixture of crushed ice in water for rapid cooling of the sample.
2. Using the Vacutainer system, draw two sequential samples, the second

being drawn into a Thrombotect tube. The first tube serves only to clear the system of activating factors and thus may be used for other tests or discarded.

3. Remove the tube from the Vacutainer adapter first, then withdraw the needle from the patient's vein.
4. Mix the tube by gentle inversion and immediately place it in the melting ice bath.
5. After 30 minutes, remove sample tube from the ice bath.
6. Remove the rubber stopper, and centrifuge the sample at 2500 × G for 20 minutes. Centrifugation temperature may vary from 2° to 30°C. An alternate centrifugation procedure should be used if centrifugation at 2500 × G is not possible. For this procedure remove the sample tube from the ice bath after 30 minutes. Remove the stopper and rim inside of tube with a cotton swab to remove any residual blood left under the stopper. Insert a plasma separator on top of the tube, and centrifuge at 1500 × G for 30 minutes or at 1000 × G for 40 minutes.
7. After centrifugation, using a plastic pipette, carefully remove 0.5 ml of the platelet-poor plasma from approximately 1 cm below the surface.
8. Place the plasma in a plastic sample tube. Samples may be stored at 2° to 8°C for 24 hours or at −20°C for up to 3 months.

Procedure

1. Bring all reagents and specimens to room temperature before testing.
2. Number and label tubes for the performance of the test as follows: tubes 1, 2, and 3, total-count tubes (TCT) for the determination of total radioactivity; tubes 4 and 5, nonspecific binding (NSB); tubes 6 through 15 for the 5 standards (0, 10, 30, 50, 100) done in duplicate; and 2 tubes for each patient sample to be tested, continuing to number in order.
3. Add 50 μl of dilution buffer into the bottom of tubes 4 and 5 (NSB).
4. Add 50 μl, in duplicate, of the standards into the bottom of the appropriately labeled tubes. Dilution buffer is used as the 0 ng/ml standard.
5. Add 50 μl of patient's platelet-poor samples into the bottom of the appropriately labeled tubes.
6. Pipette 250 μl I-125 PF_4 reagent solution into the lower portion of all tubes. Cap tubes 1 through 3 (TCT) and set aside.
7. Pipette 250/μl dilution buffer into the lower portion of tubes 4 and 5 (NSB).
8. Pipette 250 μl PF_4 antiserum into tubes beginning with 6.
9. Mix all tubes, except TCT tubes, on a vortex mixer for 3 to 5 seconds.
10. Incubate tubes at room temperature for 2 hours.
11. Pipette 1 ml ammonium sulfate solution into all tubes, except TCT tubes.
12. Mix tubes on the vortex mixer for 3 to 5 seconds, then allow to stand for at least 10 minutes, but not longer than 60 minutes, before centrifugation.
13. Centrifuge all tubes, except TCT, at room temperature at 1000 to 1500 × G for 20 minutes.

14. Decant the supernate, and determine the net radioactivity in each tube. Take an average of the two determinations of each sample to make calculations.

Results

1. Calculate the percentage of I-125 PF$_4$ bound to antiserum in the ammonium sulfate precipitate.

$$\frac{\text{cpm Standard or Unknown} \times 100}{\text{Average cpm TCT}} = \% \text{ Bound}$$

2. Using linear graph paper, plot the percentage bound for each PF$_4$ standard on the vertical axis vs the corresponding labeled concentration for each vial on the horizontal axis. Using the 5 points, draw the best-fit smooth curve.
3. Determine the concentration of PF$_4$ in unknown samples from this curve.

Expected Value: 0 to 10.4 ng/ml

References

Package Insert—Platelet factor 4 (PF$_4$) RIA Kit. North Chicago, IL, Abbott Laboratories, 1980.

Green LH, Seroppean E, and Handlin RI: Platelet activation during exercise-induced myocardial ischemia. N Engl J Med *302*:193, 1980.

Handlin RI, McDonough M, and Lesch M: Elevation of platelet factor four in acute myocardial infarction: measurement of radioimmunoassay. J Lab Clin Med *91*:340, 1978.

Technique for Measurement of B-TG

Equipment

1. Gamma scintillation counter.
2. Refrigerated centrifuging capable of 2000 × G and with a horizontal head.
3. Crushed ice and water bath.
4. Precision pipettes—50, 200 and 500 μl size.
5. Vortex mixer.
6. Assay tubes—12 × 75 mm polystyrene tubes, round bottomed.

Reagents (Reagents are included in the B-TG/RIA Kit from Amersham Corporation)

1. Standard B-TG (human) in buffer (freeze-dried) vials (5). Reconstitute each vial of standard with 0.5 ml distilled water. Allow to dissolve at room temperature and invert gently to mix. The exact value of each standard is stated on the vial.
2. I-125 B-TG (human) contains up to 2 μCi I-125 per vial. Reconstitute vial with 10 ml distilled water.
3. Anti-B-TG (rabbit) contains antiserum sufficient to bind at least 40% of 0.5 ng B-TG. Reconstitute with 10 ml distilled water.
4. Ammonium sulfate solution (3.3 M).
5. Blood collecting tubes contain anticoagulant and antiplatelet agents.

Collection and Preparation of Samples

1. Place blood-collecting tubes provided in the kit in the crushed ice and water bath to cool.
2. Using the two-syringe technique with a plastic syringe and a 20-gauge × 1 inch needle, collect about 3 to 4 ml blood.
3. Immediately after blood collection, remove needle from syringe and gently add 2.5 ml of blood to a precooled, labeled sample tube.
4. Replace the cap on tube and mix by gently inverting the tube several times. Immediately place tube of blood back in the cooling bath. The blood sample must be mixed with the anticoagulant and antiplatelet reagent and cooled as rapidly as possible, following sample collection.
5. Allow sufficient time for specimen to cool (approximately 30 minutes).
6. Centrifuge the sample at 1500 to 2000 × G and 2 to 4°C for 30 minutes. Centrifugation must be carried out within 3 hours after sample collection.
7. After centrifugation, carefully remove the top 0.5 ml of plasma to a separate labeled polystyrene tube. Use a pipette with disposable plastic tip.
8. The sample for assay may be stored at room temperature for up to 24 hours; at 2 to 5°C for 1 week; or up to 4 weeks at −20°C.

Procedure

1. Number and label the polystyrene test tubes in order, 2 for each of the five standards and 2 for each patient sample to be tested.
2. Starting from the lowest standard to the highest, place 50 μl of the reconstituted standards into each of 2 appropriately labeled tubes. (Tests are to be done in duplicate.)
3. Place 50 μl of plasma from each patient into each of 2 appropriately labeled tubes.
4. Add 200 μl of the B-TG I-125 solution into each assay tube.
5. Add 200 μl of the anti-B-TG serum into each assay tube and vortex each for 3 to 5 seconds.
6. Incubate the assay tubes at room temperature for 1 hour. Place parafilm over the rack of tubes during this incubation period.
7. Add 500 μl of ammonium sulfate solution to the assay tubes and immediately vortex mix each tube thoroughly.
8. Centrifuge the tubes for 10 to 15 minutes at room temperature at 1000 to 1500 × G.
9. Place the tubes in decantation racks and carefully pour off supernatants, making sure the precipitate remains undisturbed at the bottom of the tubes.
10. Keeping the tubes inverted, place them on a paper towel to drain for 5 minutes.
11. Gently touch the rims of the tubes with paper tissues to remove any liquid remaining before returning tubes to an upright position.
12. Count the precipitates in a gamma counter. Count for either 1 or 2 minutes: Calculate results as counts per minute (cpm).

Results

1. Using the linear graph paper, plot a curve of I-125 counts for the first tubes of the 5 standards versus the concentration stated on each standard vial (counts on vertical axis and concentration on horizontal axis).
2. Plot the points for the duplicate tubes of the standards and draw a smooth curve through the mean of the duplicate points.
3. Using the mean of the duplicate points for each patient sample assayed, determine the B-TG level from the standard curve.

Expected Value: 15 to 70 ng/ml.

References

Package Insert—Beta-Thromboglobulin (B-TG) RIA Kit. Arlington Heights, IL, Amersham Corp, 1977.
Smith RC, et al: B-Thromboglobulin and deep vein thrombosis. Thromb Haematol (Stutt) 39:336, 1978.

DETECTION OF PLATELET ANTIBODIES
(Inhibition of Clot Retraction)

General Principles

Damage to 90% or more of the platelets in freshly collected blood due to their interaction with an antibody or a drug-antibody complex prevents clot retraction. Preincubation of serum and platelet-rich plasma with free magnesium ions permits complement activity but not coagulation. This increases the sensitivity of the test.

Technique

Equipment and Reagents

1. Glass test tubes (12 × 75) for performing clot retraction tests.
2. Calcium chloride (0.1 M).
3. Magnesium chloride (0.1 M).
4. EDTA (5%).
5. Drugs to be tested (if indicated). Quinidine or quinine sulfate (1 mg/ml). A 200 mg tablet may be crushed, dissolved in 100 ml distilled water at 37° for 30 minutes, and the insoluble material removed by centrifugation. Hydrochlorothiazide (saturated solution) Sulfasoxizole (0.2 mg/ml).

Preparation of Blood Samples

1. Draw 5 ml blood from a patient suspected of having antibodies and allow it to clot. Incubate the clotted sample for 2 hours at 37°C and centrifuge. Remove serum and place in a glass test tube.
2. Draw 15 ml blood from an ABO-compatible normal donor and add 10 ml to a tube containing 0.3 ml of 5% EDTA. Place the remainder in a tube and allow it to clot, handling it in the same way the patient's sample is handled. Centrifuge the EDTA tube for 10 minutes at 1000 rpm and remove 2.0 ml of the platelet-rich plasma. This may be adjusted to a final concentration of 200,000/mm³ by diluting it with platelet-poor plasma obtained by further centrifugation of the EDTA tube for 10 minutes at 3000 rpm.

Procedure

1. Add 0.1 ml of patient's serum to each of 2 glass test tubes.
2. Add 0.02 ml magnesium chloride to each tube.
3. If drug solutions are to be tested, label tubes and add 0.2 ml drug solution to one tube and 0.2 ml distilled water to the other.
4. Set up two more tubes containing normal control serum in the same way.
5. Add 0.3 ml platelet-rich plasma to each tube and gently mix.
6. Incubate the tubes at 37°C for 1 hour.
7. Following incubation, add 0.02 ml calcium choride to each tube and allow clot to form. "Flick" the tip of each tube to loosen the clot and incubate for an additional hour at 37°C.
8. Observe for clot retraction. Free fluid can be measured semiquantitatively after careful removal of the clots.
9. If the patient's platelet count has returned to normal, the test may be done on 0.4 ml patient's platelet-rich plasma.

Interpretation

Failure of retraction of clots in tubes that contain patient's serum when retraction is normal in clots formed in the absence of patient's serum suggests the presence of platelet antibodies. If retraction is abnormal only in the presence of the drug solution, then the antibody is drug-dependent. Complement-fixing antibodies such as those found in quinidine and quinine thrombocytopenia or in post-transfusion purpura are most likely to give positive results, but the test is capable of detecting some isoantibodies also.

Reference

Aster RH: Detection of Antiplatelet Antibodies Inhibition of Clot Retraction. *In* Hematology. Edited by WJ Williams, et al. New York, McGraw-Hill, 1972, p. 1417.

CHAPTER 6

Evaluation of the Intrinsic Pathway

WHOLE-BLOOD CLOTTING TESTS

General Principles

The whole-blood clotting time (WBCT) is a function of the combined factors that favor coagulation and those that inhibit it. It is a gross test of the intrinsic pathway (Figure 6-1) and is not satisfactory as a screening procedure in the study of hemorrhagic diseases. Results are influenced by many external factors. The clotting time is increased by (1) increasing the volume of blood, (2) increasing the diameter of test tubes, and (3) decreasing the temperature. The time is shortened by (1) tilting and (2) the presence of tissue thromboplastin that may be introduced from a traumatic venipuncture. With strict adherence to specific conditions, it is possible to maintain reproducible results, but even when this is accomplished, the usefulness of the test is limited by its lack of sensitivity to most mild coagulation disorders. In patients with hemophilia A, the whole-blood clotting time usually is not prolonged unless the concentration of factor VIII is less than 1%; however, circulating anticoagulants nearly always produce significant prolongations. The test is most useful for comparative studies in monitoring heparin therapy, but is time-consuming when clotting times are prolonged. It is often included as part of the prothrombin consumption test.

The ground-glass clotting time (GGCT) and the activated clotting time (ACT) are much less affected by external factors and have fairly good sensitivity for detecting patients with mild disorders of coagulation. They are more practical than the whole-blood clotting time for monitoring patients who are receiving heparin therapy, especially during open heart surgery. They have the particular advantage of requiring a much shorter time to complete than the whole-blood clotting time. Also, they require little specific equipment and no reagents. They can be conveniently done at the patient's bedside, and their accuracy is increased by the use of a 37°C electric heating block or a portable automated instrument.

Whole-Blood Clotting Time

Procedure

1. Using the two-syringe technique, draw 5 ml blood into a plastic syringe.
2. Immediately place 1 ml blood in each of 3 glass tubes, and place these

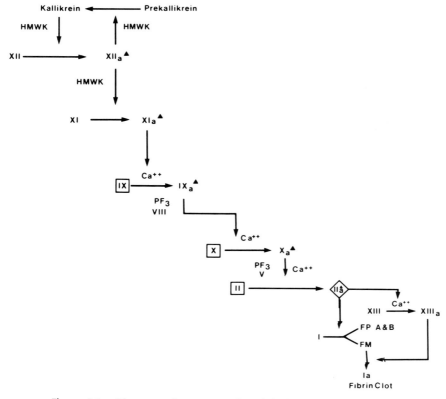

Figure 6-1. Diagrammatic representation of the intrinsic pathway.

tubes in the 37°C water bath or electric heating block. Start a stopwatch when the blood is placed in the third test tube.

3. Tilt the first tube every minute until it can be inverted with no flow of blood down the side of the tube. Then tilt the second tube until the blood in it clots, and the third tube in a similar manner.

4. Report the clotting time of the third tube.

5. Tubes may be left in the water bath for the prothrombin consumption test and for observation of clot lysis.

Normal Values: 7 to 15 minutes.

References

Lee RL, and White PD: A clinical study of the coagulation time of blood. Am J Med Sci 145:495, 1913.
Sirridge MS: Pitfalls in the performance and interpretation of laboratory studies for hemorrhagic disorders. Am J Med Tech, 30:399, 1964.

Ground-Glass Clotting Time

Equipment

1. Particles of ground glass are obtained by crushing discarded glassware with a mortar and pestle. The fragments should vary in size from fine dust

to particles about 1 mm in diameter. Type 070 Super-Brite beads (Potter's Industries, Inc., Carlstad, NJ) may also be used.

2. 37°C water bath or electric heating block.

Procedure

1. Place enough glass (about 75 mg) in 3 glass test tubes to cover the bottom of the tubes, and place these in the 37°C water bath or electric heating block.
2. Draw blood in a plastic syringe and place 1 ml in each of the 3 tubes.
3. Quickly and firmly seal the tubes with rubber stoppers.
4. Immediately invert the first tube, starting a stopwatch at the same time.
5. Rapidly invert the 3 tubes in sequence until a clot appears. The end point is the formation of a solid clot that adheres to the bottom of the test tube; however, when the clotting time is considerably prolonged, the end point may be noted as the formation of a large clot that slides down the tube when it is inverted.
6. The clotting time of each tube is noted to the nearest 5 seconds, and the average of the three results is reported.

Normal Values: 90 to 140 seconds.

Reference

Hoffman ME, and Synder A: The ground-glass clotting time. Cleveland Clin Quart 33:107, 1966.

Activated Clotting Time

Equipment

1. Dry Vacutainer tube.
2. Vacutainer tube evacuated to draw 2 ml and containing 12 mg siliceous earth (Becton-Dickinson No. 6522).
3. 37°C water bath or electric heating block. Portable automated instruments are also available (Thermolyne ACT-stat Incubator, Thermolyne Corp., Dubuque, IA, or Hemochron, Int. Technidyne Corp., Edison, NJ).

Procedure

1. Draw 1 ml or more of blood into a dry Vacutainer tube by venipuncture. (This tube aspirates any tissue thromboplastin that has entered the needle.)
2. With the needle still in the vein, remove the tourniquet and replace the initial tube with the Vacutainer tube containing the siliceous earth (pre-warmed to 37°C). When blood appears in the tube, start the timer. Alternatively, blood could be drawn into a plastic syringe, using the two-syringe technique, and 2 ml transferred to the clotting-time tube.
3. When the tube has filled, invert it a few times to mix and place it in the 37°C water bath or electric heating block.
4. At 1 minute, and at 5-second intervals thereafter, withdraw the tube and

tilt it. Time to the nearest 5 seconds the appearance of the first unmistakable clot.

Normal Values: 71 to 101 seconds.

References

Forman WB, and Bayer G: A simplified method for monitoring heparin therapy at the bedside: the activated whole blood clotting time. Am J Hematol *11*:277, 1981.
Hattersley PG: Activated coagulation time of whole blood. JAMA *196*:150, 1966.
Hattersley PG: Progress report: the activated coagulation time of whole blood (ACT). Am J Clin Pathol 66:899, 1976.
Stenbjerg S, Berg E, and Albrechtser OK: Heparin levels and activated clotting time (ACT) during open heart surgery. Scand J Haematol *26*:281, 1981.
Stenbjerg S, Berg E, and Albrechtser OK: Evaluation of the activated whole blood clotting time (ACT) in vitro. Scand J Haematol *23*:239, 1979.

PLASMA CLOTTING TESTS

General Principles

Plasma clotting tests also measure the intrinsic pathway, but there are several important differences between these procedures and those in which whole blood is tested. Plasma clots much more rapidly than does whole blood, and this is an indication that significant changes must occur in blood from the time of drawing until the plasma is separated and tested. Since blood is mixed with calcium-binding anticoagulants to obtain plasma, it is apparent that the changes that occur do not require calcium. They are primarily the time-consuming contact-activation reactions. The wide range of plasma recalcification times in normal subjects is partially due to varying degrees of contact activation, thus the manner of drawing and handling blood is of importance in standardizing any such procedure. Temperature and pH also influence the rate of clotting, and other changes in clotting activity occur when plasma is stored. Platelet-poor plasma clots much more slowly than does platelet-rich plasma, indicating that the rate of plasma clotting is also partially dependent on platelet activity.

The sequence of events in the clotting of plasma after calcium is added is diagrammatically shown in Figure 6-2. Over half the time is required for further contact activation and the next longest period is that of so-called thromboplastin formation, a process that is influenced by platelet activity. Thus, the two most time-consuming reactions are most affected by the way in which blood is collected and handled. The time required for the conversion of prothrombin to thrombin and the thrombin-fibrinogen reaction is relatively short and has less influence on the overall result. It seems logical that maximizing contact activation and platelet activity, both of which are difficult to keep constant under the usual circumstances of blood collection, should make it possible to use plasma recalcification techniques in the detection of abnormalities in the plasma clotting factors that participate in the intrinsic pathway. This is the rationale behind the difference in the three plasma clotting procedures: plasma recalcification time, partial thromboplastin time (PTT), and activated partial thromboplastin time (APTT).

The *plasma recalcification time* may be performed on platelet-rich plasma or platelet-poor plasma. When a platelet-rich sample is tested, all aspects of the intrinsic

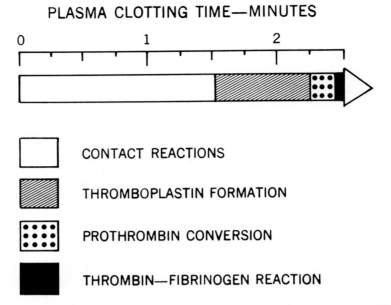

Figure 6-2. Blood coagulation viewed as a series of reactions of different time relations. (From Biggs R, and MacFarlane RG: Human Blood Coagulation, 3rd Ed. Courtesy of Blackwell Scientific Publications, 1963.)

pathway are evaluated, including the contribution of platelet factor 3. Such a test is especially sensitive to inhibition by the lupus anticoagulant, which apparently inhibits phospholipid. When platelet-poor samples are tested, the clotting times are much longer and the test measures the intrinsic pathway coagulation reactions,

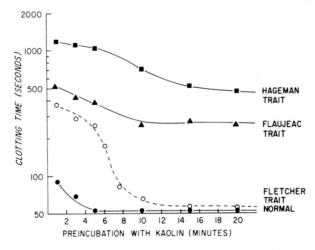

Figure 6-3. Effect of preincubation with kaolin on the APTT of Flaujeac plasma. The results obtained with normal, Hageman trait, and Fletcher trait plasmas are also given. (From Wuepper KD, et al: Flaujeac Trait: deficiency of human plasma kininogen. J Clin Invest 56:1663, 1975. Used by permission of the American Society for Clinical Investigation.)

which occur much more slowly in the absence of normal amounts of platelet phospholipid. Most coagulation tests (PT, APTT, factor assay, and others) are done on platelet-poor plasma; the recalcification test on platelet-rich plasma is done less often because it requires additional processing of the plasma. The APTT and PTT are more sensitive and reproducible than the recalcification time when testing for abnormalities of coagulation factors.

The *partial thromboplastin time* (PTT) is a modification of the plasma recalcification procedure. In the PTT, a platelet substitute is added and platelet activity is not tested for. Since the test measures the intrinsic pathway, it cannot detect a deficiency of factor VII, which has a necessary function only in the extrinsic pathway. The test involves the same problems as those of the plasma recalcification time, with the exception of the ones that are due to variations in platelet numbers. The addition of a partial thromboplastin reagent gives maximum platelet activity and a shorter clotting time than that obtained with the simple addition of calcium to platelet-poor plasma. Such reagents, however, do not standardize contact activation, and the problems still remain of careful collection and the changes that occur in plasma on standing. These may be minimized by using plastic syringes and test tubes and by performing the test promptly after the withdrawal of the blood. Results should always be questioned if the plasma has stood over 2 hours, even if it has been refrigerated. Also, the particular anticoagulant used may influence the results to some degree. A control plasma should always be run with each group of tests, although this is not always completely comparable if the control is a commercial product, obtained and handled in a different way.

The PTT is not sensitive to minor coagulation-factor deficiencies, and since the activities of so many factors are measured together, overall prolongation may be masked by elevated levels of one or more individual factors or active intermediates. Occasionally, an abnormal PTT may be the only abnormality of coagulation found, in which case its importance is equivocal and should be evaluated by further testing. The PTT is much more likely to be prolonged with defects of the contact factors and factors VIII and IX than with abnormalities of factors that act later in the coagulation cascade. In patients whose prothrombin times are prolonged because they are receiving coumarin-type oral anticoagulant drugs, the PTT tests often remain within the normal range and the relationship of the two test values is variable (Table 6-1). The

TABLE 6-1. Comparison of Prothrombin Times and Partial Thromboplastin Times in 20 Patients on Oral Anticoagulants

Prothrombin Time (in seconds)	PTT* (in seconds)
15-23 (17 samples)	68-97
19	108
23	105
30	101

* Using Thrombofax (normal <100 seconds).

plasma recalcification time of platelet-rich plasma is much more likely to show changes comparable to those of the prothrombin time.

Another important point to remember is that the final clotting time in the PTT test is affected by the manner and speed of tilting, which should be gentle and slow. Automatic instruments vary in methodology, and in some no agitation occurs at all. Results with different instruments, therefore, are not strictly comparable with each other or with results obtained by manual methods. The need for comparable controls with all tests cannot be over-emphasized, since reagents may not always be stable and may contain unknown activator or inhibitor substances.

The *activated partial thromboplastin time* (APTT) is a further modification of the plasma recalcification time, in which an activator substance is added to the platelet substitute in order to maximize and thus standardize contact activation. It gives even shorter clotting times and a narrower range of average values and has greater reliability and sensitivity to coagulation-factor deficiencies.

Table 6-2 gives a comparative evaluation of the plasma recalcification time of platelet-poor plasma (PPP), the partial thromboplastin time, and the activated partial thromboplastin time in detecting reduced concentrations of factor VIII. The information was obtained by making successive dilutions of a standard normal plasma with

TABLE 6-2. Comparison of Plasma Clotting Procedures in the Detection of Deficiency of Factor VIII

	Recalcification Time (in seconds)	Partial Thromboplastin Time (PTT) (in seconds)	Activated PTT (APTT) (in seconds)
Standard Normal Plasma (SNP)	152	75	52
Patient 0.5 ml } App. 50% SNP 0.5 ml	155	77	54
Patient 0.8 ml } App. 20% SNP 0.2 ml	180	97	85
Patient 0.9 ml } App. 10% SNP 0.1 ml	215	115	102
Patient (1% Factor VIII)	375	220	213

plasma from a patient with less than 1% factor VIII. The recalcification time and partial thromboplastin time did not become distinctly abnormal until the factor VIII level was less than 20%. The activated procedure was highly abnormal at the 20% level, although not at the 50% level. This would indicate that, in this situation, the activated test was the most sensitive of the three. APTT values are extremely prolonged in patients who are homozygous for deficiencies of factor XII, prekallikrein, and high molecular weight kininogen (>200 seconds); however, levels of <1% factors VIII and IX usually give values of <100 seconds.

The activated partial thromboplastin reagent is valuable for doing assay procedures for all of the contact factors as well as for factors VIII and IX. The PTT or the

APTT are preferred for mixing studies in patients who have circulating anticoagulants. Results are more reproducible than with the whole-blood clotting time or plasma recalcification time except in the case of the lupus anticoagulant, in which the plasma recalcification time of platelet-rich plasma may be the most sensitive test.

Problems in the Use and Interpretation of PTT and APTT Tests

1. Since these tests measure the combined activities of the contact factors and factors IX, VIII, X, V, II, and I, results may be falsely normal in some deficient states because of concomitant increases and decreases in different factors.
2. Both of these tests lack sensitivity to mild deficiency states of single clotting factors. Very mild deficiencies may result in normal or only slightly prolonged values. Since the activated modification appears to be more sensitive, the PTT is now rarely used.
3. Lack of sensitivity to changes produced by therapy with coumarin-type drugs makes the tests unsatisfactory as single procedures for overall screening (Table 6-1).
4. Commercial controls do not reflect the variation seen in normal individuals, and some have deliberately been prepared to provide faster clotting times than most normal samples. Abnormal controls are available from commercial sources and may permit a separation of significant abnormal test results. The significance of slight prolongation of clotting time when there is no history of bleeding and no other abnormal test results still remains unknown. Many people with such results have had uneventful surgical procedures, and may represent the "slow activator" abnormality or other abnormalities of contact activation.
5. Results of both of these tests, particularly when done on abnormal samples, may be influenced by the anticoagulant used. This was mentioned in the discussion of the partial thromboplastin time. Times tend to be longer with oxalate than with citrate and shorter with acid-citrate. See Table 6-3 for a comparison of results on a single abnormal plasma when anticoagulated with two different anticoagulants and tested with three different reagents. With all reagents, the acid-citrate anticoagulant gave appreciably shorter times.

TABLE 6-3. Comparison of Activated Partial Thromboplastin Times
of a Single Abnormal Plasma Collected with Different
Anticoagulants and Tested with Different Reagents

Anticoagulant	Reagent 1 (Ellagic Acid Activated) (in seconds)	Reagent 2 (Ellagic Acid Activated) (in seconds)	Reagent 3 (Kaolin Activated) (in seconds)
3.8% Sodium citrate	56.5	68.5	105.0
Acid-citrate	42.8	57.2	64.0
Lyophilized control	38.9	37.5	38.0

6. A significant lack of uniformity exists among activated partial thromboplastin reagents, much more so than among thromboplastin reagents. At least three different types of activating substances are used in available commercial reagents—kaolin, micronized silica, and ellagic acid. These activators have different properties and some plasmas are not activated to the same degree with all activators. It is known that patients with a deficiency of prekallikrein will have prolonged APTT tests when kaolin or micronized silica is used as an activator, but normal results with ellagic-acid-activated reagents.

7. Recommended incubation times differ with different reagents and procedures. As shown in Table 6-4, the test results of five different plasmas showed progressive but variable shortening, with increasing periods of activation. It was also noted that two different lots of the same reagent gave different results with the same control plasma. The length of the incubation times is particularly important in abnormalities of the contact factors. As shown in Figure 6-3, incubation of prekallikrein (Fletcher factor)-deficient

TABLE 6-4. Incubation Time and the Results of the Activated Partial Thromboplastin Time Test Using an Ellagic Acid-Activated Reagent

	Incubation Time (in seconds)				
Reagent* Lot No. 1	30	60	120	180	300
Control	56.5	50.2		43.8	42.5
Patient					
No. 1	66.0	59.9	49.2	44.5	41.0
No. 2	56.0	50.0	44.5	40.2	34.0
No. 3	43.0	38.5	36.0	33.0	29.2
No. 4	50.0	42.2	43.9	41.2	36.8
No. 5	55.0	50.0	44.5	40.2	34.0
Reagent* Lot No. 2					
Control	60.0	52.0		46.2	41.5

* Activated Thrombofax.

plasma with kaolin for 10 minutes normalized the APTT. Little correction occurred after prolonged incubation of plasmas deficient in factor XII (Hageman) and high molecular weight kininogen (Flaujeac factor).

8. Thromboplastin contamination resulting from poor venipuncture technique represents a common problem for this test. The acceleration of clotting produced by these tissue products may mask deficiencies that ordinarily would produce a prolonged value. This can be prevented in most instances by careful use of the two-syringe technique.

9. Other variables are hematocrit, temperature, pH, and calcium concentration.

10. Partial thromboplastin tests are not completely satisfactory for monitoring heparin therapy but are preferable to the whole-blood clotting time (Lee

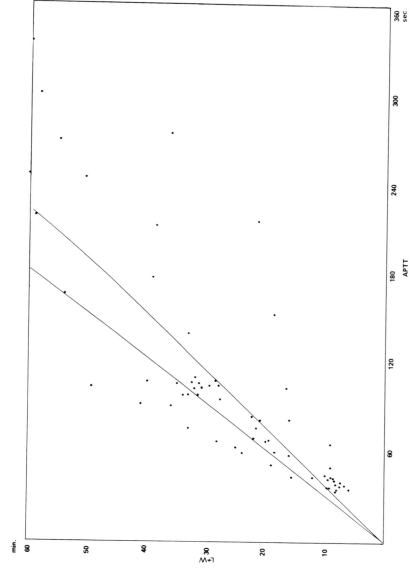

Figure 6-4.   Correlation of the APTT in seconds and the Lee and White whole-blood clotting times in minutes on 50 separate samples from patients receiving heparin therapy. The area between the two lines represents good correlation.

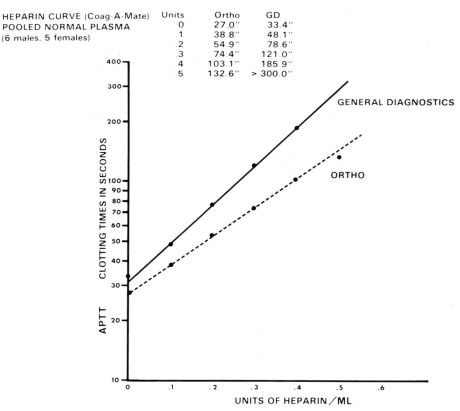

HEPARIN CURVE (Coag-A-Mate)	Units	Ortho	GD
POOLED NORMAL PLASMA	0	27.0″	33.4″
(6 males, 5 females)	.1	38.8″	48.1″
	.2	54.9″	78.6″
	.3	74.4″	121.0″
	.4	103.1″	185.9″
	.5	132.6″	> 300.0″

Figure 6-5. Heparin curves made by testing samples of pooled normal plasma to which measured amounts of heparin were added. The heparinized samples were tested with two APTT reagents which gave different results.

and White). With low to moderate concentrations of heparin, the correlation between these tests is good, but this is not true with higher concentrations (Figure 6-4). Also, considerable variation exists in the sensitivity of different APTT reagents to the concentration of heparin in plasma, as shown in Figure 6-5.

11. Circulating anticoagulants occur occasionally and prolong both partial thromboplastin times, so they must always be considered and tested for in evaluating results. Addition of the plasma recalcification time done on platelet-rich plasma may be helpful in such situations.

References

Entes K, LaDuca FM, and Tourbaf KD: Fletcher factor deficiency, source of variations of the activated partial thromboplastin time. Am J Clin Pathol 75:626, 1981.

Sirridge MS: Pitfalls in the performance and interpretation of laboratory studies for hemorrhagic disorders. Am J Med Tech 30:399, 1964.

Triplett DA, Harms CS, and Koepke JA: The effect of heparin on the activated partial thromboplastin time. Am J Clin Pathol 70:556, 1978.

Plasma Recalcification Time

Reagents

1. Sodium citrate (3.8%), sodium oxalate (0.1 M) or acid-citrate solution.
2. Calcium chloride (0.025 M).
3. Normal plasma (a fresh sample collected in the same manner as the test sample should be used).

Procedure

1. Add 4.5 ml blood to 0.5 ml anticoagulant solution and mix. If platelet-rich plasma is to be tested, collect the blood by the two-syringe technique in a plastic syringe and place it in a plastic tube. Siliconized Vacutainers can also be used, if this is the second tube. Blood for platelet-poor plasma can be collected by the regular Vacutainer technique.
2. Centrifuge blood samples for 10 minutes at 1000 rpm to obtain platelet-rich plasma or for 10 minutes at 3000 rpm to obtain platelet-poor plasma. The test may be run on either sample or both. The plasma should be stored in plastic tubes and should not stand longer than 2 hours.
3. Place a tube of calcium chloride solution in the 37° C water bath to warm.
4. Place 4 glass tubes in the 37° C water bath and add 0.2 ml of normal plasma to the first tube.
5. Blow into the plasma 0.2 ml calcium chloride solution and start a stopwatch.
6. Allow the tube to stand in the water bath for 60 seconds; then remove it, tilting gently no more than once per second. Stop the watch when the fibrin web forms. Repeat the test with the second tube. If platelet-poor plasma is being tested, allow the tube to remain in the water bath for 100 seconds before starting the tilting.
7. Test the patient's plasma in exactly the same manner.

Normal Value: Platelet-rich plasma 120 to 160 seconds; Platelet-poor plasma 160 to 200 seconds.

Interpretation

This test measures the intrinsic pathway. The time varies inversely with the platelet concentration, so the time of centrifugation is critical and the result must be compared to a normal plasma handled in the same manner. Patients with lupus anticoagulants may show striking prolongation of the result when platelet-rich plasma is tested.

Partial Thromboplastin Time

Reagents

1. Sodium citrate (3.8%), sodium oxalate (0.1 M), or acid-citrate solution.
2. Partial thromboplastin reagent.
3. Calcium chloride (0.025 M).

4. Normal plasma (commercial control-plasma made by the manufacturer of the PTT reagent may be used).

Procedure

1. Add 4.5 ml blood to 0.5 ml anticoagulant solution and mix. Vacutainers can be used if this is the second tube drawn.
2. Centrifuge the blood immediately for 10 minutes at 3000 rpm and remove the plasma, refrigerating it until use. The plasma should be stored in a plastic tube and should not stand longer than 2 hours.
3. Place an aliquot of the normal plasma and a tube of calcium chloride solution in the 37°C water bath to warm.
4. Place 0.1 ml partial thromboplastin reagent into 4 glass tubes and allow to warm at 37°C for 3 minutes.
5. Pipette 0.1 ml normal plasma into one of the tubes containing reagent and mix by tapping gently. Incubate the mixture for 30 seconds.
6. Blow into the mixture 0.1 ml calcium chloride solution and start a stopwatch.
7. Allow the tube to stand in the water bath for 60 seconds and then remove it, tilting gently not oftener than once per second. Stop the watch when a fibrin web forms. Repeat the test with the second tube.
8. Test the patient's plasma in the same manner in duplicate.

Normal Value: Less than 100 seconds.

References

Langdell RD, Wagner RH, and Brinkhous KM: Effect of antihemophilic factor on one-stage clotting tests. J Lab Clin Med 47:637, 1953.
Rodman NF, Barrow FM, and Graham JB: Diagnosis and control of the hemophilioid states with the partial thromboplastin (PTT) test. Am J Clin Path 29:525, 1958.

Activated Partial Thromboplastin Time

Reagents

1. Sodium citrate (3.8%), sodium oxalate (0.1 *M*), or acid-citrate solution.
2. Activated partial thromboplastin reagent.
3. Calcium chloride solution (0.025 *M*).
4. Normal plasma (commercial control-plasma made by the manufacturer of the APTT reagent may be used).

Procedure

1. Add 4.5 ml blood to 0.5 ml anticoagulant solution and mix. Vacutainers can be used if this is the second tube drawn.
2. Centrifuge the blood immediately for 10 minutes at 3000 rpm and remove the plasma, refrigerating it until use. Do not allow it to stand longer than 2 hours.
3. Place an aliquot of calcium chloride solution in the 37°C water bath to warm.

4. Pipette 0.1 ml activated partial thromboplastin reagent into the desired number of glass tubes and place in the water bath. Allow to warm at least 1 minute.

5. Add 0.1 ml normal plasma to the first tube. Mix well and allow to incubate at 37°C for 5 minutes, agitating occasionally. Do not allow the incubation time to exceed 5 minutes.

6. Blow in 0.1 ml calcium chloride solution and start a stopwatch.

7. Allow the tube to remain in the water bath for 20 seconds, and then remove it, tilting gently not more than once per second. Stop the watch when a fibrin web forms. Repeat the test with a second tube.

8. Test the patient's plasma in the same manner in duplicate.

9. It is possible to start the incubation of successive tubes at 2-minute intervals, thus utilizing the 5-minute incubation period that is necessary for each tube.

10. (Optional) If the clotting time of the test plasma is prolonged for unknown reasons, the procedure should be repeated with 10- and 20-minute incubation times. It is also sometimes useful to try a different APTT reagent. Prekallikrein-deficient plasmas give normal values with ellagic acid-activated reagents.

11. (Optional) If prolonged incubation does not correct a prolonged APTT, the procedure should be repeated with 0.1 ml of a mixture made of 0.2 ml patient's plasma and 0.2 ml normal plasma. Further studies can include testing a mixture of 0.4 ml patient's plasma with 0.1 ml normal plasma (20% normal plasma).

12. Several types of automated and semiautomated instruments are satisfactory for performing this test and are preferred if multiple samples are to be tested.

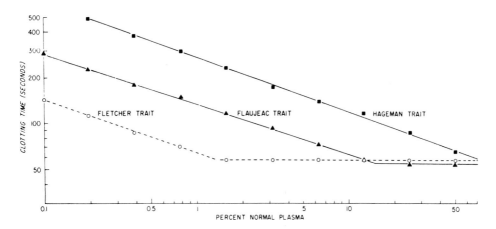

Figure 6-6. Correction of Flaujeac plasma by normal plasma. A dose-related response was given by normal plasma in concentrations less than 12.5%. The dose-dependent correction of Hageman trait and Fletcher trait plasmas is shown for comparison. (From Wuepper K, et al: Flaujeac trait: deficiency of human plasma kininogen. J Clin Invest 56:1663, 1975. Used by permission of The American Society for Clinical Investigation.)

Interpretation

The accepted range of normal values must be determined for each reagent system and end-point device. Prolonged incubation significantly shortens the APTT of pre-kallikrein (Fletcher factor)-deficient plasma, but not that of other factor-deficient plasmas. If a prolonged test value is corrected by mixing with a 20% volume of normal plasma as suggested in No. 11, the abnormality is most likely due to a deficiency, and the differential APTT or appropriate factor assays should be done. Figure 6-6 shows the marked variation in factor concentrations required for correction of the APTT in plasmas deficient in the contact factors. If the APTT of mixtures of patient and normal plasma is intermediate between the two values or as long as that of the patient, a circulating anticoagulant should be suspected and tested for. If the APTT is to be used for monitoring heparin therapy, a heparin-control curve should be made for the reagent system and end-point system that are being used.

References

Wuepper KD, Miller DR, and Lacombe MJ: Flaujeac trait deficiency of human plasma kininogen. J Clin Invest 56:1663, 1972.
Hattersley PG, and Hyse D: The effect of increased contact activation time on the activated partial thromboplastin time. Am J Clin Pathol 66:479, 1976.
Koepke JA: The partial thromboplastin time in the CAP survey program. Am J Clin Pathol 63:990, 1975.

Differential Activated Partial Thromboplastin Time

General Principles

This differential test need be done only when the regular test is prolonged and the test value is corrected by mixing 1 part normal plasma with 4 parts patient's plasma.

Reagents

1. Adsorbed plasma reagent (source of factors I, V, VIII, XI, and XII), (page 207), or commercially available as Adsorbed Plasma Reagent.
2. Serum reagent (source of factors IX, X, XI and XII), (page 215), or commercially available as Serum Reagent.
3. All other reagents are those used in the APTT.

Procedure

The test is conducted in the same manner as the APTT (page 124), except for step 5, which is altered as follows:

Make the following mixtures:
1. 0.1 ml normal plasma and 0.4 ml patient's plasma.
2. 0.4 ml normal plasma and 0.1 ml adsorbed plasma reagent.
3. 0.4 ml normal plasma and 0.1 ml serum reagent.
4. 0.4 ml patient's plasma and 0.1 ml adsorbed plasma reagent.
5. 0.4 ml patient's plasma and 0.1 ml serum reagent.

Add 0.1 ml each mixture to 0.1 ml activated thromboplastin reagent and incubate at 37°C for 5 minutes with occasional agitation.

TABLE 6-5.   Use of the Differential APTT and PT in the Diagnosis of Isolated Coagulation-Factor Deficiencies

| Patient's Original Time | | APTT | | PT | | | Deficiency Indicated |
APTT	PT	Adsorbed Plasma Reagent	Serum Reagent	Adsorbed Plasma Reagent	Serum Reagent	V-Deficient Plasma	
A	N	C	NC	—	—	—	VIII
A	N	C	C	—	—	—	XI, XIII, HMWK, or prekallikrein
A	N	NC	C	—	—	—	IX
A	A	—	—	C	NC	C	I
A	A	—	—	C	NC	NC	V
A	A	—	—	NC	C	C	X
A	A	—	—	NC	NC	C	II
N	A	—	—	NC	C	C	VII

N = normal time; A = abnormal time; C = corrected time relative to clotting time of normal plasma + reagent; — means not applicable; NC = time not corrected.

Interpretation (Table 6-5)

1. If the mixture of normal and patient's plasma in tube 1 gives a normal result, this suggests a coagulation factor deficiency and the testing should continue. Lack of correction suggests a circulating anticoagulant.
2. If the addition of adsorbed plasma reagent to the patient's plasma in tube 4 gives a clotting time that approximates that of the mixture in tube 2, factor VIII is probably deficient. (Deficiency of factor V or I is ruled out by a normal prothrombin time.)
3. If the mixture of serum reagent and patient's plasma in tube 5 approximates the result obtained in tube 3, factor IX is probably deficient. (Factor X deficiency is ruled out by a normal prothrombin time.)
4. Correction of the abnormal test result by both reagents indicates a probable deficiency of factor XI, XII, prekallikrein, or high molecular weight kininogen.

Example

		Adsorbed Plasma		Serum	
Normal Plasma	42''	No. 2	43''	No. 3	45''
Factor VIII deficient Plasma	84''	No. 4	45''	No. 5	97''
Factor IX deficient Plasma	80''	No. 4	97''	No. 5	47''
Factor XI deficient Plasma	215''	No. 4	52''	No. 5	45''

5. When the APTT and PT are done on the same specimen, it is possible to be more precise in determining coagulation-factor abnormalities (Figure 6-7). The presence of clinical bleeding is also useful in differential diagnosis.
6. If the APTT is only minimally prolonged, the PTT may give more clear-cut results with differential substitution.

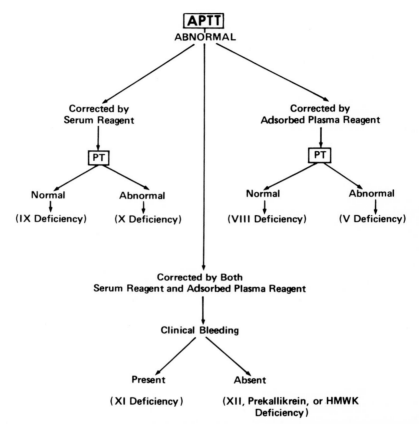

Figure 6-7. Use of the results of the differential APTT and the PT in the investigation of a patient with an abnormal APTT.

Reference

Biggs R, and Douglas AS: The thromboplastin generation test. J Clin Path 6:23, 1953.

Preparation of a Heparin Control Curve for Use with the APTT

General Principles

Responses of patients to heparin are highly variable. In studies using the APTT, it has been found that some patients resist the anticoagulant effect at concentrations of 1 U/ml plasma, while others have delayed clotting at concentrations of only 0.2 U/ml. Repeated studies on a single patient at a given time, however, seem to show a consistent response. It is apparent, therefore, that the APTT reflects the anticoagulant effect rather than the heparin concentration. The same type of variable response is also seen when the thrombin time test is used. It is possible, however, to construct a satisfactory heparin-control curve for use with either of these tests by using a pool of several plasmas in an effort to measure an average relationship of heparin concentration to anticoagulant activity. The ideal procedure would be to construct a heparin-control curve for each patient being treated, prior to institution of heparin therapy, and to utilize this to determine the patient's heparin concentration at a given time.

Reagents

1. Pool of fresh platelet-poor citrated plasmas from at least 6 donors.
2. Barbital-buffered saline.
3. Activated partial thromboplastin reagent (curve should be prepared with the same reagent that is regularly used to test patient's samples).
4. Calcium chloride solution (0.025 M).
5. Heparin sodium 10 U/ml. (Dilute heparin 1000 U/ml 1:100 with barbital-buffered saline, and use the same source as that used therapeutically in the hospital.)
6. Semilog graph paper.

Procedure

1. Prepare 5 dilutions of the 10 U/ml heparin solution as follows:

	Heparin (10 U/ml)		Barbital-Buffered Saline	Final Concentration (U/ml Plasma)
(1)	0.1 ml	+	0.9 ml	0.1
(2)	0.2 ml	+	0.8 ml	0.2
(3)	0.3 ml	+	0.7 ml	0.3
(4)	0.4 ml	+	0.6 ml	0.4
(5)	0.5 ml	+	0.5 ml	0.5
(6)	1.0 ml	+	—	1.0

2. Place 0.9 ml pooled plasma in each of 6 numbered test tubes. Add 0.1 ml of each dilution of heparin to a corresponding tube.
3. If preparing a curve for use with the activated partial thromboplastin time test, test each sample of heparinized plasma in duplicate by adding 0.1 ml activated partial thromboplastin reagent and allowing it to activate 5 minutes at 37°C; determine clotting time from the addition of 0.1 ml calcium chloride.
4. Using semilog graph paper, plot the points with the clotting times on the ordinate (log scale) and the heparin concentrations on the abscissa (linear scale). The resulting curve should approximate a straight line between values of 0.1 and 0.5 U/ml (Figure 6-5).

Interpretation

The activated partial thromboplastin time of the heparinized samples should relate to the heparin concentrations in a manner similar to that given in Figure 6-5.

ONE-STAGE ASSAY METHOD FOR ACTIVITY OF CONTACT FACTORS AND FACTORS VIII AND IX

General Principles

The principle of bioassay has been successfully applied to the activated partial thromboplastin time, permitting the specific and acceptably quantitative measurement of individual coagulation factors. A test system lacking a single coagulation factor is established. Various calculated amounts of the missing factor are supplied to the system, and their corrective effect is observed. The unknown or test plasma is then applied to the system in like manner. The degree of correction achieved by the unknown plasma is compared with that achieved by plasma of known concentration.

When clotting time is plotted against plasma concentration, the resulting curve has a reversed S-shape and is flat at each end. If the plasma concentration is plotted on the logarithmic scale on semilog paper, the mid-portion of the curve is virtually linear and has sufficient slope to permit discrimination. The assay procedure described here employs plasma concentrations that normally fall on the sensitive, linear portion of the coagulation-activity curve. At this critical level, differences in clotting time assume quantitative significance and can be directly related to the amount of available assay factor.

Because of its relative simplicity, a one-stage procedure is of practical use in the clinical laboratory. Authorities on coagulation have generally accepted the technique as a valid means of measuring specific-factor activity in plasma. Some authorities, however, believe that it cannot be applied to the assay of coagulation activity in other biologic materials such as factor concentrates.

This basic technique can theoretically be used to assay any coagulation factor that takes part in the APTT reaction. It is most useful for the assay of factors VIII and IX, but can also be used to assay factors XII, XI, prekallikrein, and high molecular weight kininogen (HMWK), if such factor-deficient substrates are available. Factors X, V, and II are more easily measured by the one-stage assay which utilizes the prothrombin time.

The one-stage assay procedure is one of the most sensitive tests presently available to the general laboratory worker.

Technique

Reagents

1. Sodium citrate (3.8%), sodium oxalate (0.1 M), or acid-citrate solution.
2. Calcium choride solution (0.025 M).
3. Activated partial thromboplastin reagent.
4. Normal reference plasma. Commercial reference-plasma with known factor levels or a pool of fresh plasma from at least three normal adults can be used. The pool should be centrifuged twice before use.
5. Factor-deficient plasmas: (page 213). These may be obtained from patients with known deficiencies and are available from several sources. (Lyophilized from General Diagnostics, Morris Plains, NJ; Helena Laboratories, Beaumont, TX; Dade, Miami, FL; Fresh-frozen from George King Bio-Medical Inc., Overland Park, KS.)

Procedure

The basic procedure is the same for all of the factors (VIII, IX, XI, XII, prekallikrein, HMWK); only the deficient substrate is different. The described procedure is for a tilt-tube method, but automatic instrumentation can also be used.

Collection of Patient's Plasma

1. Obtain blood from the patient by means of the two-syringe technique, using Vacutainers or plastic syringes. Add 4.5 ml patient's blood to 0.5 ml anticoagulant solution.
2. Mix and centrifuge immediately for 10 minutes at 3000 rpm.
3. Remove plasma and store in an ice bath or at refrigerator temperature. It should be tested within 2 hours.
4. Frozen samples can be tested if the normal curve is made from a frozen plasma pool.

Normal Curve

1. Reconstitute a vial of commercial reference-plasma, or use a freshly collected pool of normal plasmas. Use a frozen plasma pool if a frozen sample is being tested.
2. Make serial dilutions of the normal reference plasma from 1:5 to 1:320 in buffered saline in the following way, mixing each tube well before transferring contents.
   a. Pipette 0.8 ml buffered saline into tube 1, and 0.5 ml into tubes 2 through 7 (Table 6-6).

TABLE 6-6. Preparation of Test Dilutions for Reference Plasma in the One-Stage Assay for Factor VIII or Other Factors

Tube	1	2	3	4	5	6	7
DIL	1:5	1:10	1:20	1:40	1:80	1:160	1:320
% of Factor	100.0%	50.0%	25.0%	12.5%	6.25%	3.25%	1.5%
Buffer	0.8 ml	0.5 ml	0.5 ml	0.5 ml	0.5 ml	0.5 ml	0.5 ml
Reference plasma	0.2 ml						
Mix and transfer	0.5 ml	0.5 ml	0.5 ml	0.5 ml	0.5 ml	0.5 ml	

   b. Pipette 0.2 ml normal reference plasma into the first tube and mix.
   c. Transfer 0.5 ml from tube 1 into the second tube and mix. Continue this process through tube 7. Use a different pipette for each transfer.
3. Reconstitute or thaw enough factor-deficient plasma to assay the dilutions of the normal reference plasma and the patient's plasma (approximately 2 ml or 2 vials), and pool.
4. Transfer 5.0 ml calcium chloride to a test tube and place in 37°C water bath.

5. Into a plain glass test tube add:
   0.1 ml factor-deficient plasma.
   0.1 ml of 1:5 dilution normal reference plasma.
   0.1 ml activated partial thromboplastin reagent.
7. At the end of the 2-minute incubation, blow 0.1 ml prewarmed calcium chloride into tube. Simultaneously, start stopwatch. Mix and return to water bath for approximately 45 seconds. Remove and gently tilt at the rate of once per second, while observing the clot. Duplicate determinations are performed on each dilution, and they should agree within ±2 seconds.
8. Repeat the procedure (steps 5, 6, and 7) for each of the 7 normal reference plasma dilutions.
9. Calculate the average clotting time of each dilution. Plot results on 2-cycle log-log graph paper as follows: Place plasma concentration on the abscissa, beginning with 1% at the left and proceeding to 100%. Plot the clotting times of the 7 concentrations of the normal reference plasma on the ordinate.
10. Draw the best observed straight line through these points. This is the normal activity curve.

1:5	Dilution =	100.00% activity
1:10	Dilution =	50.00% activity
1:20	Dilution =	25.00% activity
1:40	Dilution =	12.50% activity
1:80	Dilution =	6.25% activity
1:160	Dilution =	3.12% activity
1:320	Dilution =	1.50% activity

Patient's Plasma Results

1. Make a 1:5 and a 1:10 dilution of patient's plasma and test in the same way as for the reference plasma. (If the 1:5 dilution gives a clotting time that is longer than the 1:320 dilution of the normal reference plasma, it is unnecessary to test the 1:10 dilution). Read the percentage of the factor being tested from the abscissa of the graph by finding the point where the time obtained for the 1:5 dilution of patient's plasma intercepts the normal curve.
2. Read the results of the 1:10 dilution in the same manner, multiplying the percentage of activity by 2. (If the 1:5 dilution gives a value of over 100%, read the value from the 1:10 dilution and make and test a 1:20 dilution).
3. Take an average of results obtained. If factor VIII-deficient plasma is used, the results will be a percentage of normal of factor VIII, and if plasma deficient in factor IX, XI, XII, prekallikrein, or high molecular weight kininogen is used, the results will be a percentage of normal of factors IX, XI, XII, prekallikrein, or high molecular weight kininogen.

Normal Range: 50 to 150% of normal.

Interpretation

The interpretation of assay results is usually straightforward; however, as in all coagulation procedures, strict technical control is required. The specimen should be processed as soon as possible, and in any case, within 2 to 3 hours. Dilutions should be tested within 30 minutes of the time they are made. A normal activity curve must be prepared for each day's assay.

If a severely deficient plasma is being studied, it may be apparent from the prolonged clotting time of the highest concentration that no interpolation will be possible. In other words, the activity of the unknown plasma may lie far beyond the 3.12% value of the normal activity curve. The only report that can be given in this case is that the observed activity of the test plasma is less than 1.5%. Some useful data may be obtained by testing such a plasma at concentrations greater than 20% (1:5) dilution.

It is desirable to test more than one dilution of the test plasma in order to verify the validity of the assay. This is done to show that the two curves, regardless of wide differences in activity, are parallel and, consequently, that the assay system is handling each specimen in the same manner. An unsatisfactory assay may result if either the normal reference plasma or the deficient-substrate plasma has deteriorated during storage. A normal prothrombin time gives some assurance that good factor V activity remains in these plasmas.

Another possible complication is the presence of an inhibitor in the test plasma. This might cause the two curves to converge or even to cross as a result of the increasing activity that appears to develop in the test plasma with increasing dilution of the inhibitor. Adequate knowledge of the coagulation mechanism and of the inherent idiosyncrasies of all coagulation tests should ensure proper evaluation of assay results.

A simple one-stage assay procedure of this type has numerous advantages. No great technical skill or sophisticated reagents are required. One complete assay can be carried out in approximately 1 hour. The test can be performed conveniently, since deficient-substrate plasmas are commercially available.

References

Egeberg O: Assay of antihemophilic A, B, and C factors by one stage cephalin systems. Scand J Clin Lab Invest 13:140, 1961.

Elodi S, Katalin V, and Hollan SR: Some sources of error in the one-stage assay of factor VIII. Haemostasis 7:1, 1978.

Kocoshis TA, and Triplett DA: CAP survey results for factor VIII assays (1977-78). Am J Clin Pathol 73:346, 1979.

Addendum

Prekallikrein activity can also be measured by a synthetic-chromogenic-substrate assay procedure, but such substrates are not available at present for the other factors tested for in the APTT one-stage assay method.

Reference

Triplett DA, and Harms CS: Procedures for the Coagulation Laboratory. Chicago, ASCP, 1981 (p. 64 for prekallikrein assay).

STANDARD THROMBOPLASTIN GENERATION TEST (TGT)

General Principles

When first described, the standard thromboplastin generation test was the best procedure for evaluating the early stages of clotting, which terminate with the formation of a prothrombin converting complex (factors X_a, V, Ca^{++}, and PF_3). To perform the test, the blood specimens were first processed into three "reagents": adsorbed plasma, aged serum, and platelet concentrate. Adsorbed plasma contained the necessary factors V and VIII. (It also contained some XI and XII, as these factors are said to be "poorly adsorbed" from plasma.) Aged serum contained the necessary factors IX, X, XI, and XII. Platelets contributed phospholipid material (platelet factor 3) to the system and also contained or transported other coagulation factors. Because of the inherent qualitative and quantitative variability of platelet suspensions, it was common practice to use a platelet substitute or partial thromboplastin reagent for routine testing purposes. The use of platelet suspensions was reserved for special cases that gave strong evidence of a qualitative platelet defect.

When the three "reagents" were recombined, all the factors necessary for the conversion of prothrombin to thrombin were present. Upon addition of calcium chloride to the mixture, a powerful coagulant activity gradually developed. This coagulant activity was then monitored by performing serial prothrombin times on a normal plasma substrate, using aliquots from the "generation mixture" to initiate thrombin formation. By preparing several generation mixtures, using normal and test reagents in various combinations, it was possible to determine which reagent was defective and thus, by inference, which specific factor was affected.

The results of the thromboplastin generation test had to be correlated with the results of the prothrombin time, since deficiency of factor V or X affects both tests and deficiencies of factors VIII, IX, XI, and XII affect only the TGT. Factor VII is not involved in the intrinsic clotting mechanism and is not tested for in the thromboplastin generation test.

The TGT had its greatest usefulness in detecting severe, single-factor deficiencies. Although comparatively sensitive, it could not be absolutely relied on to detect the so-called mild deficiencies. The original investigators stated, for example, that if the factor VIII level exceeded 10%, then the TGT would probably be normal. Unfortunately, significant hemorrhagic disease is known to occur when the factor VIII levels are in the 10 to 30% range.

There were also some unavoidable technical problems. Relatively large volumes of blood were required. This was a major drawback when dealing with pediatric patients. There was no way to establish absolute status quo in the samples while tests were being performed over a relatively long period of time. Serum is especially capricious in this regard and is known to contain varying amounts of intermediate activation products long after macroscopic coagulation has occurred.

Although no special equipment or sophisticated reagents were required, the TGT demanded a great deal of laboratory time. After the plasma and serum reagents were prepared, an additional 1 to 2 hours of undivided attention was required for processing the necessary generation mixtures. This alone made performance of the test prohibitive for the small laboratory where technologists' time is a definite factor.

The TGT was long considered to be the best available diagnostic test for disorders of the initial stages of coagulation. Much of what we know about these stages has been learned from this test and its modifications. With the advent of the more specific and more sensitive factor-assay procedures, the usefulness of the TGT is now largely confined to the differentiation of "plasma" and "serum" defects. Extensive use of the TGT as a diagnostic test is no longer warranted, since most of the same information can be obtained from modifications of the simpler one-stage methods in much less time. Historically, it is of great importance.

Technique (Figure 6-8)

Reagents and Equipment

1. Sodium citrate (3.8%), sodium oxalate (0.1 M), or acid-citrate solution.
2. Calcium chloride solution (0.025 M).
3. Barbital-buffered saline.
4. Aluminum hydroxide gel or barium sulfate (page 207).
5. Partial thromboplastin reagent: diluted 1 : 10 with buffered-saline solution.
6. Two stopwatches are needed.

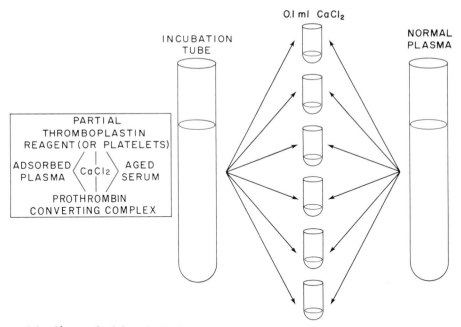

Figure 6-8. The standard thromboplastin generation test. Aliquots of partial thromboplastin reagent, adsorbed plasma, and aged serum are pipetted into the incubation tube on the left. With the addition of calcium chloride solution to this tube, the timing of the generation reaction is begun. At 1-minute intervals thereafter, for a total of 6 minutes, 0.1 ml generation mixture and then 0.1 ml normal substrate plasma are added to a tube containing 0.1 ml $CaCl_2$ solution, and the clotting time is determined.

Procedure

Preliminary Preparations

1. Obtain the following blood specimens, using the two-syringe technique. Approximately 20 ml blood are required from the normal donor and 10 ml from the patient, unless the patient's platelets are to be tested. In this case, 20 ml blood will be needed from the patient as well.

    Tube 1: Add 4.5 ml blood to 0.5 ml anticoagulant solution. Stopper and mix well by gentle inversion.

    Tube 2: Place 6 to 7 ml blood in a test tube containing 4 or 5 small glass beads. Stopper and invert until clotted. Incubate at 37°C for 4 hours.

    Tube 3: Add 9 ml blood to a plastic graduated centrifuge tube containing 1.0 ml sodium citrate solution. Stopper and mix well by gentle inversion. (Omit this preparation of a sample from the patient unless the platelets are to be tested.)

2. Process specimens from both patient and normal donor promptly, making sure that each is clearly identified. The use of a refrigerated centrifuge is recommended, but not required.

    Tube 1: Centrifuge at 2000 rpm for 5 minutes. Remove plasma. If sodium citrate anticoagulant is used, add 0.15 ml aluminum hydroxide gel to 1.5 ml plasma. Stopper and shake for 5 minutes. Centrifuge at 3000 rpm for 5 minutes. Transfer the adsorbed plasma to a clean test tube. Determine its prothrombin time. The result should be longer than 1 minute. If sodium oxalate is used as an anticoagulant, barium sulfate may be used as the adsorbent (150 mg/1.5 ml plasma), but barium sulfate cannot be used with citrated plasma. Refrigerate the adsorbed plasma until ready to perform the test. Immediately before testing, make a 1:5 dilution with buffered-saline solution (0.5 ml plasma to 2.0 ml buffered saline).

    Tube 2: After incubation of the clotted blood, rim the clot and centrifuge at 2500 rpm for 10 minutes. Remove the serum. Make a 1:10 dilution with buffered-saline solution (0.5 ml serum to 4.5 ml buffered saline). Let the diluted serum stand at least 1 hour before testing.

    Tube 3: If only normal substrate plasma is needed, centrifuge the normal donor specimen at 3000 rpm for 30 minutes. Remove the plasma and refrigerate. If platelet suspensions are desired, first centrifuge both donor and patient specimens at 1500 rpm for 5 minutes. Transfer platelet-rich plasma to clean siliconized or plastic graduated centrifuge tubes. Measure the plasma volume. Centrifuge at 3000 rpm for 30 minutes. Transfer platelet-free plasma to clean test tubes and refrigerate. Wash the sedimented platelet buttons 3 times in 5 ml buffered saline solution, resuspending the platelets by stirring with an applicator stick between each wash.

After the third wash, add fresh saline solution equivalent to one third the original plasma volume. Resuspend the platelets and refrigerate (refrigeration will produce a smoother suspension).

Performance of the Test

1. Place an aliquot of normal substrate plasma in the water bath to warm to 37°C.
2. Pipette 0.1 ml calcium chloride solution into each of the 6 glass test tubes and place in the 37°C water bath.
3. Place a 15 × 100 mm test tube (incubation tube) in the water bath, and add, in succession:
    a. 0.3 ml partial-thromboplastin reagent or normal platelet suspension.
    b. 0.3 ml normal adsorbed plasma.
    c. 0.3 ml normal serum.
    This is the generation mixture.
4. Allow the generation mixture to stand for 2 minutes.
5. Add 0.3 ml calcium chloride solution to the generation mixture and start a stopwatch immediately.
6. At 45 seconds incubation time, blow 0.1 ml generation mixture into one of the test tubes containing calcium chloride solution. At 1 minute, blow 0.1 ml of the prewarmed normal substrate plasma into the same tube and start a second stopwatch. Remove the tube from the water bath and observe for coagulation by the usual tilting method. If no clot has formed within 45 seconds, discontinue the timing and proceed to the next step.
7. Continue to sample the generation mixture at 1-minute intervals as described in step 6 for a total of 6 minutes. Record each clotting time. In a normal sample, the clotting time will be 14 seconds or less at 3 to 5 minutes after generation is begun. A clot may form in the generation mixture, but this does not affect the test results. It should be removed to avoid pipetting difficulty.
8. After the normal control system proves satisfactory, the following additional generation mixtures are prepared and tested in the same manner.
    a. Partial thromboplastin reagent + patient's adsorbed plasma + patient's serum.
    b. Partial thromboplastin reagent + normal adsorbed plasma + patient's serum.
    c. Partial thromboplastin reagent + patient's adsorbed plasma + normal serum.
    d. Mixtures containing patient's and normal platelet suspensions instead of partial thromboplastin reagent must be tested to determine platelet function.

Interpretation

1. The TGT is assumed to be normal if a clotting time of 14 seconds or less is achieved at any time during the 6-minute test period.

2. If the result is abnormal only when the patient's adsorbed plasma is used, the deficiency is presumed to be factor VIII. (Factor V deficiency is ruled out by a normal prothrombin time.)

3. If the test is abnormal only when the patient's serum is used, the deficiency is presumed to be factor IX. (Factor X deficiency is ruled out by a normal prothrombin time.)

4. If the result is abnormal when the patient's plasma and serum are used together, but normal when each is tested separately, the deficiency is presumed to be factor XI, factor XII, prekallikrein, or high molecular weight kininogen. Differentiation between these deficiencies is best made by performing individual assays using factor-specific deficient substrates. Fortunately, their occurrence is rare.

5. Circulating anticoagulants can also interfere with the early clotting reactions—most commonly, an inhibitor of factor VIII. If the TGT is abnormal, it is therefore necessary to determine whether this abnormality is due to a deficiency or to an inhibitor. If this has not already been established, it can be done most easily by testing a pre-incubated mixture of equal parts of normal and patient's plasma in the partial thromboplastin time test. It is possible, however, to test for anticoagulant activity in the thromboplastin generation test by mixing 0.15 ml patient's adsorbed plasma with 0.15 ml normal adsorbed plasma and allowing the mixture to stand at room temperature for 15 minutes. This mixture can then be used as the adsorbed plasma reagent in an otherwise normal generation mixture. The normal adsorbed plasma that is now included in the test system should provide ample factor VIII to produce normal thromboplastin generation. If the generation is not normalized, one must assume that an anticoagulant substance in the patient's plasma has inhibited the reaction. Since the activity of inhibitors of factor VIII is dependent on time and temperature, the result may be intermediate between the normal and abnormal after such brief incubation at room temperature. If this is the case, results after incubation for a period of 1 hour at 37°C should be compared to those obtained using a sample of normal adsorbed plasma that has been handled in the same way. Fortunately, such anticoagulants are not common; however, the number of patients having these has increased with the widespread use of factor concentrates, and it is extremely important that they be recognized before replacement therapy is instituted. Factor assay techniques are more specific.

6. After properly evaluating the test results, a presumptive interpretation can be made, reporting, for example, as "adsorbed plasma deficiency, presumptively, factor VIII."

Addendum

We no longer use the whole-blood screening thromboplastin-generation test or the Hicks-Pitney test because of the ready availability of factor-deficient substrates that are needed for specific assay procedures. The standard thromboplastin-generation test is presented mainly because of its historical importance.

References

Biggs R, and Macfarlane RB: Human Blood Coagulation and its Disorders, 3rd Ed. Oxford, Blackwell Scientific Publications, 1962.

Biggs R, and Macfarlane RB: Treatment of Hemophilia. Philadelphia, F.A. Davis, 1966.

Miale JB: Laboratory Medicine—Hematology, 2nd Ed. St. Louis, C.V. Mosby, 1966.

Sirridge MS, Bowman AB, and Allwin JF: A simple whole blood screening test for disorders of thromboplastin generation. Am J Clin Pathol 37:551, 1962.

ROCKET IMMUNOELECTROPHORETIC ASSAY FOR FACTOR VIII-RELATED ANTIGEN (VIIIR:Ag)

General Principle

Factor VIIIR:Ag can be measured in plasma by means of the rocket immunoelectrophoretic assay described by Laurell. This technique is based on the electrophoretic migration of an antigen through a thin gel medium containing the specific antiserum. The height of the precipitating peak depends on the concentration of the antigen in the sample and allows quantitative measurement of factor VIIIR:Ag. Such measurements are useful in the diagnosis of hemophilia A, von Willebrand's disease and in the detection of hemophilia A carriers.

Technique

Equipment

1. Power supply.
2. Electrophoresis cell with cooling coil.
3. Glass plates (2 × 3 inches).
4. Hot plate.
5. Water bath, 56°C.
6. Well cutter (Gelman Sciences Inc., Ann Arbor, MI).
7. Suction needle (Gelman).
8. Staining and rinsing tanks (Gelman).
9. Leveling table (Gelman) or any level surface.
10. Micro pipette (5 μl).

Reagents

1. Antiserum to human factor VIII (Calbiochem-Behring Corp., LaJolla, CA).
2. Agarose (must be stored in a tightly closed container).
3. Dextran T-10 (Pharmacia Fine Chemicals, Inc., Uppsala, Sweden).
4. NaCl 0.85% weight/volume (W/V).
5. Tris-barbital buffer, pH 8.8 (0.03 M): Dissolve 9.76 g sodium barbital, 2.47 g barbital and 5.87 g tris in 2 L distilled water (available as High Resolution Buffer from Gelman).
6. Protein stain (Bioware Inc., Wichita, KS): Dissolve 0.2 g of protein stain in 45 ml absolute methanol, 10 ml glacial acetic acid and 45 ml distilled or de-ionized water.

7.   Destaining solution: Mix 90 ml methanol with 90 ml distilled or deionized water and 20 ml glacial acetic acid.

Collection and Preparation of Plasma Samples

Patient

1.   Obtain blood from the patient by means of the two-syringe technique, using Vacutainer or plastic syringes. Add 9 parts patient's blood to 1 part sodium citrate, (blood anticoagulated with EDTA may be used if plasma for the standard is collected in EDTA).
2.   Mix and centrifuge for 10 minutes at 3000 rpm. If plasma is to be assayed at a later date, freeze immediately at $-30°C$ in plastic tubes. Factor VIIIR:Ag is stable for 1 year.
3.   Before assaying, prepare patient's plasma dilution, 1:1 (undiluted) and 1:2 with tris-barbital buffer.

Reference Pool

1.   Collect and prepare plasma specimens as above from at least 10 normal donors. (Do not use donors who are pregnant or taking oral contraceptives.)
2.   Pool plasmas. Plasma may be stored in aliquots at $-30°C$ and thawed when ready to use.
3.   Prepare pooled normal plasma dilutions (reference), 1:1 (undiluted), 1:2, 1:4, and 1:8 with tris-barbital buffer. The 1:1 dilution represents 100% of normal. These dilutions are used to prepare the reference curve.

Procedure

1.   Prepare a 0.9% agarose solution in tris-barbital buffer. Add to this mixture 1 g Dextran T-10 per 100 ml agarose solution. Heat the solution to the boiling point. When the solution has cleared, cool to 56°C in a water bath. A temperature above 56°C may denature the antibody.
2.   Dilute antiserum 1:5 with saline and warm to approximately 56°C.
3.   Add 0.175 ml of the diluted antiserum to each 10 ml of the agarose solution and mix gently. (The proper antiserum concentration may need adjusting, depending on the lot number.)
4.   Place the glass plates on the leveling table or on any flat, level surface.
5.   Pour about 8 ml of the agarose-antiserum mixture on each clean glass plate and distribute the mixture evenly. The temperature of the mixture must be high enough to ensure true fluidity.
6.   Allow to cool. When the gel has solidified, using a suction needle, punch a row of seven wells parallel to the 2-inch edge of the plate. Each well should be about 2.5 mm in diameter, and the wells should be approximately 4 mm apart. Four 2×3 inch glass plates may be run at one time.
7.   Label the backs of the glass plates, using a diamond-tipped pencil.
8.   In the first 5 wells on the first plate, apply 5 μl of each of the pooled normal plasma dilutions for the reference curve. Apply the 1:1 dilution to

2 wells. Add 5 μl of the 1:1 and 1:2 dilutions of the patient's plasma to wells 6 and 7 respectively.

9. On each of the remaining plates, apply at least a 1:1 and 1:2 dilution of the pooled normal plasma, and both a 1:1 and 1:2 dilution of each patient's plasma to be tested.

10. Place the plates on the bridge of the electrophoresis cell, with the wells near the cathode.

11. Fill the electrophoresis chambers with tris-barbital buffer.

    Note: If the electrophoresis chamber does not have cooling coils, use buffer that has been chilled at 4°C.

12. Cut Whatman No. 3 filter paper the length of the plates and use as wicks.

13. Soak the paper wicks in buffer solution and place along each edge of the plates and extend them down into the buffer.

14. Close the lid on the electrophoresis cell and turn on the power supply.

15. Electrophoresis conditions:
    Voltage—110 to 150 volts
    Current—10 to 12 mamp per plate
    Field strength—2 to 4 v/cm
    Electrophoresis time—14 to 18 hours (overnight)

16. After electrophoresis, rinse (soak) plates overnight in 0.85% sodium chloride in rinsing tanks.

17. Change sodium chloride and soak an additional 3 hours.

18. Soak in distilled or de-ionized water 1 hour.

19. Remove plates from rinsing tanks and cover with lint-free paper strips that have been moistened with distilled or de-ionized water. Avoid trapping air bubbles.

20. Allow plates to dry overnight at room temperature.

21. Remove paper strip and immerse the plates in the protein-stain solution for 20 to 60 minutes.

22. Remove excess stain with destaining solution. (Destain until a clear background is obtained.)

23. Dry the plates in a vertical position at room temperature.

Evaluation

1. Determine the length of the rockets to the nearest 0.1 mm by measuring the distance between the center of the application well and the end point of the rocket.

2. Construct a reference curve by plotting the length of rockets for the standard dilutions (ordinate) against their respective concentrations (abscissa), expressed as a percentage of normal (1.1, undiluted = 100%).

3. The concentration of factor VIIIR:Ag in patient's samples can be determined from the reference curve and expressed in precentage of the normal plasma pool. If the patient's antigen level is greater than 100%, use a 1:4 dilution; read the result from the graph and multiply by 4.

Normal Range: 50 to 150% of normal.

Interpretation

The greatest usefulness of this assay is in the determination of the ratio of factor VIII coagulant activity to factor VIII-related antigen (VIII:C/VIIIR:Ag). In hemophilia A, this ratio is usually less than 0.1. In hemophiliac carriers, the ratio is usually near 0.5. The use of the factor VIII:C/VIIIR:Ag ratio has been shown to discriminate 57 to 90% of obligate carriers from a normal group of females. Because of the lack of precision of this procedure, the World Health Organization has recommended that the activity and antigen determinations be done three times for each subject and that the median of the three outcomes be taken. Such results must also be related to those from a reference group of significant size studied in the same laboratory.

In von Willebrand's disease (type I), the ratio is about 1.0, with a corresponding decrease in the levels of both factors VIII:C and VIIIR:Ag. The ratio is variable in types IIA and IIB of this disorder.

Addendum

Immunoradiometric assays can also be used for the measurement of factor VIIIR:Ag. The results appear to be comparable, but the tests are more complicated and required more extensive apparatus.

References

Akhmeteli MA, et al: Method for the detection of haemophilia carriers: a memorandum. Bull WHO *55*:675, 1977.

Laurell CB: Quantitative estimation of proteins by electrophoresis in agarose gel containing antibodies. Anal Biochem *13*:45, 1966.

Peake IR, et al: Carrier detection in haemophilia A by immunological measurement of factor VIII related antigen (VIIIR:Ag) and factor VIII clotting antigen (VIIIC:Ag). Br J Haematol *48*:651, 1981.

Zimmerman TS, Ratnoff DD, and Littel AS: Detection of carriers of classic hemophilia using an immunologic assay for antihemophilic factor (factor VIII). J Clin Invest *50*:255, 1971.

Zimmerman TS, Ratnoff DD, and Powell AE: Immunologic differentiation of classical hemophilia (factor VIII deficiency) and von Willebrand's disease. J Clin Invest *50*:244, 1971.

CHAPTER *7*

Laboratory Testing for von Willebrand's Disease

General agreement now exists that the basic defect in von Willebrand's disease is an abnormality or deficiency of factor VIII. Besides being essential for normal coagulation, factor VIII is also necessary for normal platelet function. For this reason, laboratory testing involves coagulation tests as well as platelet function tests and thus does not fit neatly into the chapter categories chosen for this book. In this chapter, we list all the tests that are useful in the diagnosis of von Willebrand's disease and include procedures for those tests that are not described in other chapters.

Circulating factor VIII is a complex of two different molecules with distinct functions, under separate genetic control. The component under the regulation of the X-chromosome is the smaller of the two, has the procoagulant properties, and is inactivated by human antibodies from hemophilia patients who have undergone multiple transfusions. Its procoagulant activity is referred to as factor VIII:C; but when it is measured immunologically by its reaction with specific human antibodies, it is referred to as factor VIIIC:Ag. The larger component of the complex, which is under the regulation of an autosomal gene, serves as the carrier protein. Immunologic detection using heterologous antisera measures this protein as VIIIR:Ag. When its interaction with platelets in the presence of ristocetin is measured, it is called VIIIR:RCF or VIIIR:WF. Crossed-immunoelectrophoresis testing gives information about the electrophoretic properties of this protein that are related to its function in platelet aggregation.

Figure 7-1 gives a summary of the results in the testing of two patients with clinically mild and severe von Willebrand's disease when compared to a normal subject. The patterns of ristocetin aggregation are abnormal but significantly different in the two patients, as are the thrombokinetograms and APTT values. Bleeding times, platelet retention and factor VIII:C levels are almost identical, although abnormal.

Not shown in Figure 7-1 is the often demonstrated exaggerated and prolonged increase in factor VIII:C when patients with von Willebrand's disease receive plasma or cryoprecipitates. One such patient showed an increase in factor VIII:C from 21% to 42% after receiving only 2 units of fresh frozen plasma. This level persisted for over 48 hours.

143

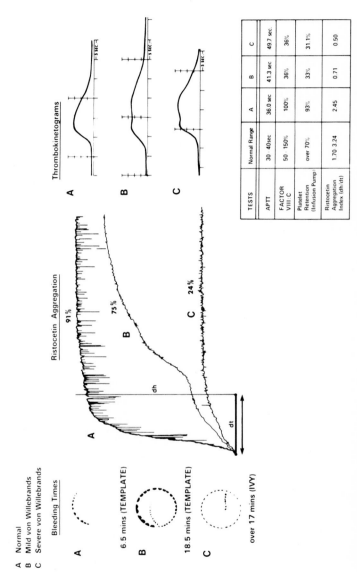

Figure 7-1. Results of bleeding times, ristocetin aggregation patterns, thrombokinetograms, APTT, factor VIII:C levels, platelet retention, and ristocetin aggregation indices in a normal patient (A) and two patients with von Willebrand's disease (B—mild) and (C—severe).

As mentioned in Chapter 2, this disorder has at least 3 variants and by the use of a group of tests that measure the various factor VIII-related activities, it is possible to distinguish these variants, as shown in Table 7-1.

The following tests are useful diagnostically:
1. Bleeding time and aspirin-tolerance test (page 71).
2. Platelet retention in glass bead columns (page 80).
3. Activated partial thromboplastin time (page 124).
4. Coagulation assay for factor VIII:C (page 130).
5. Immunologic assay for factor VIIIR:Ag (page 139).
6. Ristocetin cofactor assay for factor VIIIR:RCF.
7. Crossed immunoelectrophoresis.
8. Response of factor VIII:C levels to infusion of plasma or concentrates (pages 26 and 143).

TABLE 7-1. Tests for Factor VIII-Related Activities in the Different Types of von Willebrand's Disease

	Type I Mild → Severe	Type IIA	Type IIB
VIII:C	↓ → ↓ ↓ ↓	Variable	Variable
VIIIR:Ag	↓ → ↓ ↓ ↓	May be normal	May be normal
VIIIR:RCF	↓ → ↓ ↓ ↓		
(VIIIR:WF)		Always ↓	Variable
Ristocetin aggregation	Variably ↓	Variably ↓	↑
Crossed immunoelectrophoresis	Normal	Abnormal	Abnormal

RISTOCETIN COFACTOR ASSAY (VIIIR:RCF)

Equipment
1. Platelet aggregometer.
2. Refrigerated centrifuge.
3. Water bath, 37°C.
4. Plastic screw-cap test tubes, 16 × 150 mm.
5. Plastic centrifuge tubes.
6. Micropipettes.

Reagents
1. NaCl, 0.15 M. (A large volume is needed and can be stored at 4°C.)
2. Tris-saline buffer, pH 7.4.
3. 0.2% NaN_3 in tris-saline buffer.
4. Formaldehyde, 2%. (Dilute concentrated formaldehyde (37%) to 2% in 0.15 M NaCl.)
5. Ristocetin (Sigma Ristocetin, R-7752) dissolved in tris buffer to a final concentration of 10 mg/ml. (Store in 0.5 ml aliquots at −30°C.)

Preparation of Formalin-Fixed Platelets
1. Obtain a unit of newly expired platelet concentrate from a blood bank and warm to 37°C for 1 hour.

2. Aliquot the platelet concentrate into large plastic screw-cap test tubes and dilute with an equal volume of 2% formaldehyde. Mix gently by inversion and place at 4°C at least 18 hours.
3. Centrifuge at 4°C at 107 × G for 10 to 15 minutes. Transfer the supernatant, which contains platelets, into plastic centrifuge tubes.
4. Centrifuge at 2500 × G at 4°C for 10 minutes. Pour off the supernatant.
5. Resuspend platelets (as gently as possible) in approximately 50 volumes of cold 0.15 M NaCl and centrifuge at 4°C at 2500 × G for 10 minutes.
6. Pour off supernatant and repeat this washing procedure two more times.
7. After the third and final wash, resuspend the platelets in tris buffer, containing 0.02% NaN_3. Adjust the platelet count to 200,000 per cu mm.
8. Store in 4 ml aliquots at 4°C until ready for use. Resuspend gently before using.
   Note: Formalin-fixed platelets are commercially available from Bio/Data Corp., Hatboro, PA.

Collection of Sample and Reference Pool

1. Obtain blood from patient by means of the two-syringe technique, using Vacutainers or plastic syringe. Add 9 parts whole blood to 1 part anticoagulant (sodium citrate 3.8%). Centrifuge for 10 minutes at 3000 rpm and remove plasma.
2. For reference pool, collect and prepare plasma specimens as above from at least 10 normal donors and pool together. (Women who are pregnant or taking oral contraceptives should not be included.) Pooled plasma may be frozen in aliquots.

Procedure

1. Prepare serial dilutions of the reference pool in tris buffer (1:2, 1:4, 1:8, 1:16). The 1:2 dilution represents 100% of normal.
2. Prepare 1:2 and 1:4 dilutions of the patient's plasma to be tested.
3. Pipette 0.25 ml fixed-platelet suspension and 0.25 ml buffer into an aggregometer cuvette and mix thoroughly. This is the reference blank.
4. Pipette 0.4 ml fixed-platelet suspension into a second aggregometer cuvette. Add 0.05 ml of the 1:2 reference-pool dilution into the cuvette and incubate for approximately 2 minutes at 37°C.
5. Add a stir bar to cuvette and place it in the aggregometer.
6. Set the 0 and 100% baselines according to manufacturer's instruction for the aggregometer being used.
7. When the 0% baseline is stable, add 0.05 ml ristocetin and note this point on the chart.
8. Observe aggregation on the chart recorder until the reaction appears complete.
9. Repeat steps 4 through 8 for the 1:4, 1:8, and 1:16 dilutions.
10. Repeat steps 4 through 8 for the 1:2 and 1:4 dilutions of patient's plasma.

Calculation

1. Measure the slope of the aggregation curves for each of the different dilutions. Slope = the change in optical density per minute on the steepest part of the curve, as measured down the middle of the curve and expressed in millimeters (see Figure 5-13, page 96).
2. On log-log paper, plot the percentage activity on the horizontal axis and the slope, in mm, on the vertical axis for each of the four standard dilutions.
3. Draw a "best fit" line through the points.
4. Determine the percentage activity for both dilutions of the patient's plasma by locating the points where the slope values intersect the standard curve. Average the results.

Normal Range: 50 to 150% of normal.

References

Allain JP, et al: Platelets fixed with paraformaldehyde: a new reagent for assay of von Willebrand factor and platelet aggregating factor. J Lab Clin Med *85*:318, 1975.

Olson JD, et al: Evaluation of ristocetin–Willebrand factor assay and ristocetin-induced platelet aggregation. Am J Clin Pathol *63*:210, 1975.

Ramsey R, and Evatt BL: Rapid assay for von Willebrand's factor activity using formalin-fixed platelets and microtitration technique. Am J Clin Pathol *72*:996, 1979.

FACTOR VIII-RELATED ANTIGEN-CROSSED IMMUNOELECTROPHORESIS

Equipment

1. Electrophoresis cell with cooling coil.
2. Power supply.
3. Glass plates (2 × 3 inches).
4. Hot plate.
5. Water bath, 56°C.
6. Leveling table set (Gelman) or any level surface.
7. Staining and rinsing tank.
8. Micropipettes, 2 μl and 75-100 μl.
9. Surgical blade, Bard Parker, No. 11.
10. Strip of plastic, approximately 6 inches long and 4 mm thick.

Reagents

1. Antiserum to human factor VIII (Calbiochem-Behring Corp., LaJolla, CA).
2. Agarose (must be stored in a tightly closed container).
3. Protein stains (Bioware, Inc., Wichita, KS): Dissolve 0.2 g of protein stain in 45 ml absolute methanol, 10 ml glacial acetic acid, and 45 ml distilled or de-ionized water.
4. Evans blue dye: 1% Evans blue dye diluted 1:4 in 20% bovine albumin (Sigma). (May be stored at 4°C.)

5.   NaCl, 0.85% W/V.
6.   Buffers
   a.   Dissolve by heating 5.52 g barbital and 30.8 g sodium barbital in 2 L distilled or de-ionized water. Adjust the pH to 8.6. Use this solution in electrophoresis chamber.
   b.   Dilute 50 ml of the buffer in "a" with 100 ml distilled or de-ionized water. Divide the diluted buffer into 2 parts. Adjust one part to pH 9.5 (for first dimension) and the other part to pH 8.6 (for second dimension).

Collection and Preparation of Plasma Samples

1.   Obtain blood from the patient by means of the two-syringe technique, using Vacutainers or plastic syringes. Add 4.5 ml patient's blood to 0.5 anticoagulant solution (sodium citrate 3.8%).
2.   Mix and centrifuge for 10 minutes at 3000 rpm. If plasma is to be assayed at a later date, freeze immediately at $-30°C$ in a plastic test tube.
3.   Recentrifuge plasma immediately before testing for 10 minutes at 3000 rpm.
4.   A normal plasma pool and a mixture of normal and patient's plasma should be tested simultaneously.

Procedure

First Dimension (Figure 7-2)

1.   Prepare an 0.9% agarose solution in diluted buffer, pH 9.5. Boil solution to dissolve, and cool in water bath to 56°C.
2.   Place plastic strip on a glass plate parallel to and approximately 0.5 inches from the 5-inch edge.
3.   Pipette 2 ml agarose onto the smaller section of the plate and distribute evenly up to the corners and edges.
4.   Allow to cool, then carefully slide away the plastic strip.
5.   The plates may be used immediately or may be stored in a moist chamber at 4°C for up to 2 weeks.
6.   Cut a well for the sample in the agarose with the surgical blade. Well must be large enough for 80 μl of sample.
7.   Mix 75 μl of sample plasma with 2 μl of the Evans blue dye marker and apply to sample well.
8.   Do the same with a pooled normal plasma that is run for comparison.
9.   Run in electrophoresis chamber with undiluted buffer, pH 8.6. The anode should be opposite the sample well. If electrophoresis cell does not have cooling coils, use buffer that has been chilled to 4°C.
10.   Electrophorese or run plates in chamber at 3.5 mamp per plate until marker dye has migrated exactly 6.5 cm from center of the sample well.
11.   After electrophoresis, keep plates in moist chamber until immediately before pouring and running second dimension to avoid drying out the agar.

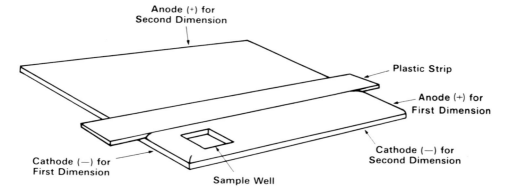

Anode (+) for
Second Dimension

Plastic Strip

Anode (+) for
First Dimension

Cathode (−) for
Second Dimension

Cathode (−) for
First Dimension

Sample Well

Figure 7-2. Preparation of plates for factor VIII-related antigen crossed immunoelectrophoresis (first and second dimension).

Second Dimension (Figure 7-2)

1. Prepare an 0.9% agarose solution in diluted buffer, pH 8.6. Boil solution to dissolve and cool in water bath to 56°C. A temperature above 56°C may denature the antibody.
2. Add antibody to the agar so that a 1 : 200 dilution of antibody in agarose is obtained (example, 100 μl antibody to 20 ml agarose). Mix well. The proper antiserum concentration may need adjusting, depending on the lot number.
3. Remove plate from moist chamber and cut a thin slice off the gel of the *first* dimension plate with the surgical blade to make the edge straight before the second dimension is poured.
4. Pipette 5 ml of the agarose mixture onto the remaining portion of plate. First and second dimension must be in direct contact. Agarose must be even and run up to the corners and edges of plates.
5. When the agarose has solidified, the second dimension is electrophoresed in the same chamber as the first dimension (plates are turned 90°). Use Whatman No. 3 filter paper as wicks.
6. Electrophorese at 5 mamp per plate for 16 hours (overnight).

Washing and Staining

1. Wash plates in 0.85% NaCl twice, 3 hours each washing.
2. Soak plates in distilled or de-ionized water for 1 hour.
3. Remove plates from rinsing tank and cover with a wet piece of Whatman No. 3 filter paper. Avoid trapping air bubbles.
4. Allow plates to dry overnight at room temperature.
5. Remove filter paper and immerse the plates in the protein-staining solution for 20 minutes.
6. Immerse plates in destaining solution for 30 minutes. Remove plates and rub the backs with a paper towel to remove excess stain.
7. Allow to dry in a vertical position at room temperature.

Evaluation

1. Measure the distance of migration from the center of sample well (d_0) to the beginning of the antigen-antibody reaction (d_1) and to the end of the fastest migrating fraction (d_2). Record results in millimeters.
2. Compare the pattern with that of the normal plasma pool run at the same time. (Example of mean value for 10 normal plasmas: d_0-d_1 = 6 mm, d_0-d_2 = 27.5 mm, d_1-d_2 = 22.1 mm).
3. If an abnormal pattern is detected in the test sample, the mixture of patient and normal plasma pool should be helpful.

Interpretation

Measurements are variable in patients with von Willebrand's disease, but tend to be similar within family groups. Usually, the mobility is faster than normal, and the end of a peak may not reach baseline. If plasma mixtures from abnormal and normal subjects are tested, 2 peaks will usually be seen.

References

Laurell CB: Antigen-antibody crossed electrophoresis. Anal Biochem *10*:358, 1965.
Sultan Y, Simeon J, and Caen JP: Electrophoretic heterogeneity of normal factor VIII/von Willebrand protein and abnormal electrophoretic mobility in patients with von Willebrand's disease. J Lab Clin Med *87*:185, 1976.
Triplett DA, and Harms CS: Procedures For The Coagulation Laboratory. Chicago, IL, ASCP, 1981.

CHAPTER 8

Evaluation of the Extrinsic Pathway

PROTHROMBIN TIME

General Principles

The end point of both the intrinsic and extrinsic pathways is the formation of a fibrin clot. Actually, the two pathways unite with the activation of factor X, and the remaining reactions are often referred to as the common pathway.

The prothrombin time (PT) is the best screening test for the reactions of the extrinsic pathway. It measures the "extrinsic" activation of factor X by the tissue thromboplastin–factor VII complex and the resulting common pathway reactions (Figure 8-1). When the PT is prolonged, the deficient factor or factors can usually be identified by a series of substitutions in the procedure. Assay values for deficient factors may be obtained through the use of plasma dilutions and specific factor-deficient plasma in the PT test in much the same way as factors VIII, IX, and the contact factors are assayed by the activated partial thromboplastin time (APTT).

The PT measures the clotting time of plasma in the presence of an optimal concentration of tissue extract. It measures to some degree the activity of five different factors: factor I (fibrinogen), factor II (prothrombin), factor V, factor VII, and factor X. Paradoxically, it is least sensitive to deficiency of the substrate factor II (prothrombin), usually showing only about a 2-second prolongation when the level of the factor is reduced to 10% of normal. The following is a list of conditions or situations in which the PT may be prolonged.

1. Congenital deficiencies of factors I, II, V, VII, and X. With afibrinogenemia, no clot forms in the test. In hypofibrinogenemia, the clotting time is not prolonged unless the level of fibrinogen is less than 80 mg%; however, dysfibrinogenemia may significantly prolong the time. Homozygous defects of factors V, VII, and X give prolonged times (>70 seconds), but in the heterozygous states (20% to 65% of normal), the prolongation is only 1 to 3 seconds. Approximately 30% of normal concentration of any of these 3 factors is sufficient to maintain a maximal rate of thrombin formation. All these conditions are rare.

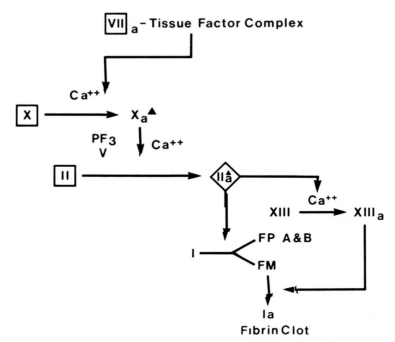

Figure 8-1. Diagrammatic representation of the extrinsic pathway.

2. Acquired multiple deficiencies of factors II, VII, and X are common and
    may be associated with coumarin-type anticoagulant therapy, paren-
    chymal liver disease, and deficiency of vitamin K.
3. Heparin, when given exogenously, acts as an anticoagulant, and a single,
    large intravenous dose prolongs the PT for varying lengths of time up to 4
    to 6 hours. For this reason, it is important to draw a specimen for determi-
    nation of the PT before heparin therapy is started, or at least 6 hours after a
    large intravenous dose has been given. Prothrombin times can be used to
    evaluate the extrinsic pathway in patients receiving continuous-infusion
    heparin therapy if the APTT is not over twice normal.
4. Circulating anticoagulants may produce prolongation of the PT as well as
    the whole-blood clotting time and the activated partial thromboplastin
    time (APTT). Isolated acquired factor V anticoagulants, which affect both
    the PT and the APTT, have been found in a few patients particularly in the
    postoperative period.
5. Disseminated intravascular clotting with associated fibrinolysis may cause
    decreases in many coagulation factors. Also, fibrin degradation products
    (FDP), which can act as anticoagulants, may be formed from the proteo-
    lysis of fibrinogen or fibrin and may prolong the PT moderately.
6. Dysproteinemias, including amyloidosis, may result in prolongation of the
    PT.

Normal plasma has a prothrombin time of 10 to 12 seconds, depending on the
activity of the particular tissue thromboplastin being used. Because the single most

EVALUATION OF THE EXTRINSIC PATHWAY   **153**

important variable in the test is the tissue thromboplastin, it is important to use the same product all the time and to run both normal and abnormal control plasmas with each set of determinations. Automated techniques usually give shorter times than tilt-tube methods. No two tissue extracts can be relied on to give the same reading with an abnormal plasma, although the normal control time in the two instances may be identical. This fact is demonstrated in Table 8-1.

TABLE 8-1. Prothrombin Times of Various Plasmas with Different Tissue Extracts

Plasma Score	Prothrombin Times (seconds)				
	Saline Extract of Human Brain	Acetone Extract of Human Brain	Difco	Simplastin	Acuplastin
Normal Control	15	15	15	15	15
Patient 1	36	29	35	30	30
Patient 2	40	35	45	35	36
Patient 3	39	33	38	34	29
Patient 4	41	35	38	34	29
Patient 5	29	24	25	24	21
Patient 6	54	36	44	36	32
Patient 7	31	26	26	21	20
Patient 8	17	18	21	22	20

Houghie, C: Fundamentals of Blood Coagulation in Clinical Medicine. (Courtesy of McGraw-Hill Book Co., 1963.)

Another problem is the decision as to what constitutes a normal plasma. The standard normal plasmas that are commercially available are prepared by pooling normal human plasmas under artificial conditions. If a freshly collected plasma or a pool of fresh plasma is to be used, the same donor or donors should be used regularly, since there is some variation in the prothrombin times of an unselected group of apparently normal people. Commercially available standard normal plasmas may not accurately represent all normal plasmas. Their main usefulness is that they have been tested by the manufacturers to give a value for the normal control plasma within the established control range for the specific thromboplastin reagent and may thus serve as a check on the adequacy of the reagent used in testing. The test value does not necessarily represent 100% of normal. Abnormal control plasmas are also available and should be tested regularly to evaluate the sensitivity of the reagent to decreased levels of factors II, VII, and X.

The type of anticoagulant used has some influence on the results; however, less variation occurs if platelet-poor plasma is used and if it is kept at 4°C until tested. With sodium oxalate, factor V deteriorates more rapidly; and after 4 hours, the PT is somewhat lengthened. Citrated plasma can be used for the PT test after standing for 1 to 2 hours at room temperature, 6 to 12 hours at 4°C, and 2 to 5 days at −20°C. The most correct way to report a prothrombin time is to report the control test value and the patient's test value.

In the investigation of an unexpected prolongation of a prothrombin time test, initial studies should include a repeat test on a new sample from the patient and, if the result is still abnormal, mixing studies with normal plasma. If correction does not occur with the mixing procedures, a circulating anticoagulant should be tested for. When an abnormal test value is corrected, particularly with a small volume of normal plasma, the next step should be to add various corrective reagents (such as adsorbed plasma, serum, and aged plasma) in order to determine which factor is deficient (see the discussion of differential prothrombin time, later in this chapter). When a single deficiency exists, results are usually clear-cut, but with multiple deficiencies there may be some confusion.

Differentiation of single factor VII and factor X deficiencies is possible because factor X is an integral part of the intrinsic pathway as well as of the extrinsic clotting system, and the patient with a factor X deficiency should have not only an abnormal PT but also an abnormal APTT. Also, it is known that when Russell's viper venom (Stypven) is used as the thromboplastin reagent in a prothrombin time procedure, factor VII-deficient plasma gives a normal clotting time, whereas factor X-deficient plasma gives a prolonged clotting time. The fact that Stypven does not require factor VII for its activity thus offers a method of differentiating single deficiencies of these two factors. Multiple deficiencies are more difficult to sort out.

Technique

Reagents

1. Sodium citrate (3.8%), sodium oxalate (0.1 M), or acid-citrate solution.
2. Tissue-thromboplastin (PT) reagent. Numerous commercial preparations are available. Most of these contain calcium chloride with the tissue thromboplastin in a single reagent. All should be prepared and used according to the manufacturer's instructions.
3. Normal plasma and abnormal plasma. (Commercial control plasmas made by the manufacturer of the PT reagent may be used.)

Procedure

1. Add 4.5 ml blood to 0.5 ml anticoagulant solution and mix. Vacutainers can be used.
2. Centrifuge the blood for 10 minutes at 3000 rpm as soon as possible; remove the plasma and store it in the refrigerator unless testing is to be done immediately.
3. Pipette 0.2 ml thromboplastin–calcium chloride reagent into each of the desired number of glass test tubes and allow to warm in the 37°C water bath for at least 1 minute.
4. Warm a small amount of the plasma to be tested in the water bath for 1 minute. Plasma should not be used after standing in the water bath longer than 15 minutes.
5. Forcibly blow 0.1 ml plasma into the thromboplastin–calcium chloride mixture and simultaneously start a stopwatch. The tip of the pipette containing the plasma should be held very close to the surface of the thromboplastin reagent.
6. Quickly shake the tube and hold it in the water bath until 2 or 3 seconds before the clot is expected.

7. Wipe the tube on removing it from the water bath and tilt it rapidly in front of a good light source. Stop the watch at the first appearance of a fibrin web. An automatic clot timer may be used. Repeat the test with a second tube.

8. Run a normal and an abnormal plasma and report the results for the patient and the normal control.

9. (Optional) If the test is prolonged in a patient not known to be taking anticoagulants, the test should be repeated, using 0.1 ml of a mixture made of 0.2 ml patient's plasma and 0.2 ml normal plasma. Further studies can include testing a mixture made of 0.4 ml patient's plasma and 0.1 ml normal plasma (4 volumes patient's plasma to 1 volume normal plasma).

Normal Values: 10 to 12 seconds, depending on the thromboplastin reagent being used. The abnormal control should give consistent daily results.

Interpretation

If the addition of an equal volume of normal plasma does not produce complete correction of a prolonged PT, a coagulation inhibitor should be suspected. Correction by the addition of 1 volume of normal plasma to 4 volumes of patient's plasma suggests a coagulation-factor deficiency.

References

Koepke JA, et al: The prediction of prothrombin time system performance using secondary standards. Am J Clin Pathol 68:191, 1977.
Houghie C: Fundamentals of Blood Coagulation in Clinical Medicine. New York, McGraw-Hill, 1963.
Quick AF, Stanley-Brown M, and Bancroft FN: A study of the coagulation defect in hemophilia and jaundice. Am J Med Sci 190:501, 1935.

DIFFERENTIAL PROTHROMBIN TIME

General Principles

The only single-factor deficiency that can result in a normal APTT and prolonged PT is a factor VII deficiency. Therefore, this differential test need be done only when both the regular PT test and the APTT are prolonged and when the test value is corrected by mixing 1 part normal plasma with 4 parts patient's plasma.

Technique

Reagents

1. Adsorbed plasma reagent (source of factors I and V) (page 207), or commercially available as Adsorbed Plasma Reagent.

2. Serum reagent (source of factors VII and X) (page 215), or commercially available as Serum Reagent.

3. Factor V-deficient substrate plasma (source of factors I, II, VII, and X) (page 213).

4. Remaining reagents are the same as those used for the prothrombin time.

Procedure

This test is conducted in the same manner as the PT (page 154) except that 0.1 ml of each of the following mixtures is tested.
1. 0.1 ml normal plasma and 0.4 ml patient's plasma.
2. 0.4 ml normal plasma and 0.1 ml adsorbed plasma reagent.
3. 0.4 ml normal plasma and 0.1 ml serum reagent.
4. 0.4 ml normal plasma and 0.1 ml factor V-deficient-substrate plasma.
5. 0.4 ml patient's plasma and 0.1 ml adsorbed plasma reagent.
6. 0.4 ml patient's plasma and 0.1 ml serum reagent.
7. 0.4 ml patient's plasma and 0.1 ml factor V-deficient-substrate plasma.

Interpretation (Table 6-5)
1. If the mixture of normal patient's plasma in tube 1 gives a normal result, this suggests a coagulation-factor deficiency and testing should continue. Lack of correction suggests a circulating anticoagulant.
2. If the addition of adsorbed plasma reagent to the patient's plasma in tube 5 gives a clotting time that approximates that of the mixture in tube 2, factor V is probably deficient, although factor I could also be deficient.
3. If the mixture of serum reagent and patient's plasma in tube 6 approximates the result in tube 3, factor X and/or factor VII are probably deficient. An isolated factor VII deficiency should be considered only when the APTT is normal.
4. If only factor V-deficient-substrate plasma is corrective, factor II is probably deficient.
5. When multiple deficiencies occur, usually only normal plasma is completely corrective, although more than one reagent may be partially corrective. Factors II, VII, and X become abnormal with oral anticoagulant therapy, in which case, normal plasma and factor V-deficient-substrate plasma are both completely corrective because they supply the three missing factors. Serum reagent is partially corrective because it supplies factors VII and X; adsorbed plasma reagent is completely ineffective because it supplies factors I and V, which are not deficient.

STYPVEN (RUSSELL'S VIPER VENOM) TIME

General Principles

Stypven differs from the tissue thromboplastin used in the prothrombin time test because it does not require factor VII for its action. Therefore, the Stypven time is primarily useful in differentiating deficiencies due to factors VII and X. Ordinary correction studies using the prothrombin time cannot accomplish this because the serum reagent used in the test contains both of these factors. The Stypven time test is primarily indicated when a prolonged prothrombin time is found, which is corrected only by the serum reagent. If the Stypven time is also long, factor X is probably deficient; if the Stypven time is normal, factor VII is probably deficient. Isolated factor VII deficiency is also indicated when the APTT is normal and the PT is prolonged. Platelet factor 3 has an accelerating influence on the clotting effect of Stypven, so it is important to control the concentration of platelets present. The test is properly done on platelet-rich plasma.

Technique

Reagents

1. Sodium citrate (3.8%), sodium oxalate (0.1 M) or acid-citrate solution.
2. Russell's viper venom (Stypven, Burroughs Wellcome Co., Greenville, NC). Reconstitute according to manufacturer's specification to give a 1:10,000 solution. This may be used for 7 days after reconstitution if stored at 2 to 10°C.
3. Calcium chloride (0.025 M).
4. Normal plasma (freshly prepared commercial control-plasma may be used).

Procedure

1. Draw blood in a plastic syringe and add 4.5 ml to 0.5 ml anticoagulant solution in a plastic tube. Siliconized Vacutainers can be used.
2. Centrifuge the blood as soon as possible for 10 minutes at 1000 rpm to obtain platelet-rich plasma. Separate the plasma and store in the refrigerator in a plastic tube, unless testing is to be done immediately.
3. Mix equal parts of Stypven solution (0.5 ml) and calcium chloride (0.5 ml) and pipette 0.2 ml of the mixture into each of 4 glass test tubes in the 37°C water bath.
4. Warm a small amount of the plasma to be tested in the water bath for 1 minute. Plasma should not be used after standing in the water bath over 15 minutes. A 1:4 dilution of plasma may also be tested; this is thought to increase the sensitivity of the test.
5. Forcibly blow 0.1 ml plasma into the Stypven–calcium chloride mixture and simultaneously start a stopwatch. (An automatic clot timer may be used.)
6. Quickly shake the tube and hold it in the water bath for 8 to 10 seconds.
7. Wipe the tube on removing it from the water bath and tilt it rapidly in front of a good light source. Stop the watch at the first appearance of a fibrin web.
8. Repeat the test on the second tube and also test a normal plasma control in duplicate.

Normal Values: 14 ± seconds (undiluted plasma).

Reference

Prentice CMR, and Ratnoff OD: The action of factor V and the prothrombin-converting principle. Br J Haematol *16*:29, 1969.

Addendum

The Stypven time test may be used as a one-stage assay procedure; it has been shown to be more sensitive than the prothrombin time test when assaying for factor V.

PROTHROMBIN–PROCONVERTIN TEST

The prothrombin–proconvertin test is a modification of the prothrombin time test, in which a 1 : 10 dilution of plasma is used and an excess of factors V and I is added. Since only deficiencies of factors II, VII, and X are detected with this test, it is not as widely used a screening procedure as the prothrombin time test. It is, however, satisfactory for following patients on coumarin-type anticoagulants, although not in any way superior for clinical evaluation. Prothrombin-free bovine plasma may be used as a source of factor V and factor I (fibrinogen). Also available is Simplastin-A, which combines in one reagent thromboplastin, calcium chloride, factor V, and factor I.

Reference

Ware AG, and Stragnell R: An improved one-stage prothrombin method. Am J Clin Pathol 22:70, 1952.

ONE-STAGE ASSAY METHOD FOR FACTORS II, V, VII, AND X

General Principles

The prothrombin time is the most satisfactory test system for assay of factors II, V, VII, and X, but such a method requires substrates that are deficient in each individual factor for which a test is being made. The percentage of factor activity is determined by the degree of correction obtained when dilutions of the test plasma are added to a factor-deficient substrate as compared with results of the addition of dilutions of a normal reference plasma. Substrates for all these factors are commercially available, and some are easy to prepare artificially.

Technique

Reagents

1. Sodium citrate (3.8%), sodium oxalate (0.1 *M*), or acid-citrate solution.
2. Barbital-buffered saline.
3. Lyophilized deficient plasmas (II, V, VII, X) are available from General Diagnostics, Morris Plains, NJ; Dade, Miami, FL; and Helena Laboratories, Beaumont, TX. Fresh-frozen deficient plasmas are available from George King Bio-Medical Inc., Overland Park, KS, or can be prepared.
   a. Factor II-deficient-substrate plasma (page 212).
   b. Factor V-deficient-substrate plasma (page 213).
   c. Factor VII- and X-deficient-substrate plasma (page 213).
4. Tissue thromboplastin reagent.
5. Normal reference plasma. Commercial reference plasma with known factor levels can be used or a pool of fresh plasma from at least three normal adults.

Preparation of a Normal Reference Curve

1. To 1.0 ml normal plasma add 9.0 ml barbital-buffered saline to make a 1:10 dilution (100%).

2. Make 5 further serial dilutions (1:2, 1:4, 1:8, 1:16, 1:32) of this 1:10 diluted plasma with barbital-buffered saline (final dilutions: 1:20, 50%; 1:40, 25%; 1:80, 12.5%; 1:160, 6.25%; 1:320, 3.12%).
3. Place an aliquot (3 ml) of tissue-thromboplastin reagent in the 37° water bath to warm.
4. To 0.1 ml 1:10 (100%) dilution add 0.1 ml deficient-substrate plasma and incubate at 37° for 1 minute. Determine the clotting time by adding 0.2 ml tissue thromboplastin reagent. Repeat with a second tube and continue with each of the additional 5 dilutions.
5. Plot the clotting times in seconds against the percentage of plasma concentration on 2-cycle log-log graph paper, using the abscissa for the plasma concentrations and the ordinate for the clotting times. Construct a straight line that best fits the 6 points.

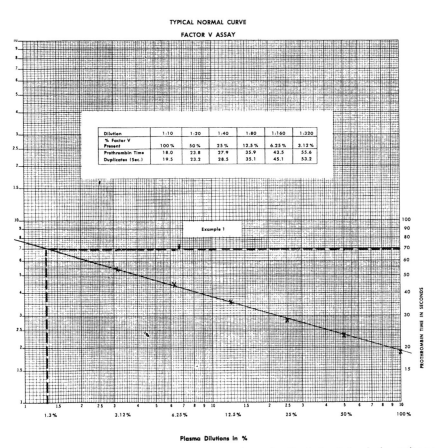

TYPICAL NORMAL CURVE

FACTOR V ASSAY

Dilution	1:10	1:20	1:40	1:80	1:160	1:320
% Factor V Present	100 %	50 %	25 %	12.5 %	6.25 %	3.12 %
Prothrombin Time Duplicates (Sec.)	18.0 19.5	23.8 23.2	27.9 28.5	35.9 35.1	43.5 45.1	55.6 53.2

Example 1

Plasma Dilutions In %

Figure 8-2.   Use of a normal factor V assay curve to determine the factor V level of a patient whose 1:10 dilution of plasma gives a clotting time of 70 seconds. Factor V activity is 1.3%. (Courtesy of Dade Division, American Hospital Supply Corporation.)

Procedure for Testing Patient Samples

1. Add 4.5 ml patient's blood to 0.5 ml anticoagulant solution and mix. Vacutainers can be used.
2. Centrifuge the blood for 10 minutes at 3000 rpm as soon as possible; separate the plasma and store in the refrigerator unless testing is to be done immediately.
3. Place an aliquot of tissue-thromboplastin reagent in the 37°C water bath to warm.
4. Dilute patient's plasma 1:10 with barbital-buffered saline. (This dilution should not be allowed to stand any longer than 30 minutes before testing.)
5. To 0.1 ml of this dilution add 0.1 ml deficient-substrate plasma (the specific substrate that is deficient in the factor to be assayed, II, V, VII, or X) and incubate at 37°C for 1 minute. Determine the clotting time by adding 0.2 ml tissue-thromboplastin reagent. Repeat with a second tube. The clotting time should be considerably longer than the normal 1:10 dilution if there is significant deficiency.
6. Read the percentage of activity directly from the normal reference curve after finding the point at which the time obtained for the 1:10 dilution of the patient's plasma intercepts the normal curve. It is well to test a further dilution (i.e., 1:20) to confirm the value. In that case, the calculated value should be multiplied by 2 and should correlate well with the value obtained from the original 1:10 dilution (Figure 8-2).

Normal Range: 50 to 150% of normal.

References

Babson AL, and Flanagan ML: Quantitative one-stage assays for factors V and X. Am J Clin Pathol 64:817, 1975.
Biggs R: Human Blood Coagulation, Haemostasis and Thrombosis, 2nd Ed. London, Blackwell Scientific, 1976, p. 231.

CHAPTER *9*

Evaluation of Fibrin Formation

THROMBIN TIME

General Principles

The end stage of both intrinsic and extrinsic pathways is the conversion of fibrinogen to fibrin by the proteolytic action of thrombin. It is possible to isolate this reaction and estimate the quantity and reactivity of fibrinogen in plasma by adding a specific amount of exogenous thrombin (bovine or human) and measuring the speed of clot formation. A standardized procedure of this kind is known as a thrombin time, and such a test may be utilized in a variety of ways. The test as it is usually performed is not very sensitive to the level of fibrinogen, being hardly affected unless the level falls below 100 mg%. When modified by using diluted plasma and an excess of thrombin, it can, however, be used to quantify fibrinogen (fibrinogen assay, Clauss). When the test is done with undiluted plasma and small amounts of thrombin, it is affected significantly by (1) alterations in the molecular structure of the fibrinogen molecule, i.e., dysfibrinogenemia; (2) the presence or absence of calcium; (3) inhibitors such as fibrinogen-fibrin degradation products and paraproteins; and (4) therapeutically administered heparin.

The thrombin time is particularly sensitive to inherited abnormalities in the structure of the fibrinogen molecule (i.e., fibrinogen Baltimore, fibrinogen Cleveland, fibrinogen Detroit). Such abnormalities result in disordered monomer polymerization and/or disordered peptide release and may thus produce variable prolongations of the thrombin time (and in some instances, the prothrombin time). When calcium chloride is added to the thrombin reagent, the reaction time is normally somewhat decreased and the end point is more obvious. Calcium is required for the activation of factor XIII by thrombin, and factor XIII$_a$ cross-links fibrin to produce a firmer and more opaque clot. In some instances, dysfibrinogenemic abnormalities are partially corrected by the presence of calcium, so the prolongation of the thrombin time with a thrombin-only reagent is much more striking than that with a thrombin-calcium reagent; therefore, the test should be performed with both reagents when such a problem is suspected. Another common abnormality in dysfibrinogenemia is increased red cell fallout in the clot retraction test (page 83).

The thrombin time is often included in a group of routine screening tests to specifically test for disorders of the thrombin-fibrinogen reaction, but it is particularly useful in testing for the presence of disseminated intravascular coagulation (DIC). In DIC, the thrombin time may be prolonged because of a decrease in fibrinogen concentration and/or the effect of fibrin degradation products (FDP) on the orderly polymerization of fibrin monomers. It is therefore useful to first measure the thrombin time and, if it is prolonged, to also measure the level of clottable fibrinogen and to test for FDP. Monoclonal paraproteins and even high levels of polyclonal immunoglobulins can also interfere with fibrin monomer polymerization and cause prolongation of the thrombin time. This effect can sometimes be decreased by testing diluted samples.

The thrombin-calcium clotting time can also be used to monitor heparin therapy, but higher than usual concentrations of calcium are required, and a heparin control curve should be made from a plasma pool to use for reference.

Technique

Reagents

1. Sodium citrate solution (3.8%).
2. Barbital-buffered saline.
3. Calcium chloride (0.025 M) or (0.1 M).
4. Thrombin solution. A stock solution may be made by adding 10 ml 50% glycerol in barbital-buffered saline to a vial containing 1000 units bovine topical thrombin (Parke-Davis, Detroit, MI), giving a concentration of 100 U/ml. This should be further diluted with barbital-buffered saline in a plastic test tube to give a plasma clotting time with normal plasma of 12 to 15 seconds. A final concentration of approximately 5 U/ml is usually satisfactory.
5. Regular thrombin-calcium solution. Instead of diluting the 100 U/ml stock solution of thrombin with buffered saline, calcium chloride (0.025 M) is used as the diluent. When the final concentration of thrombin is 5 U/ml, the thrombin time is usually 3 to 4 seconds shorter with the thrombin-calcium reagent.
6. Special thrombin-calcium solution for testing heparinized plasma. Thrombin should be diluted in barbital-buffered saline to give a concentration of 50 U/ml and then further diluted with calcium chloride (0.1 M) to provide a plasma clotting time with normal plasma of 8 to 9 seconds. A final concentration of 7 U/ml is usually satisfactory.
7. Normal plasma. (Freshly prepared commercial standard plasma of known fibrinogen concentration is best.)
   Note: A thrombin clotting time kit is available from Bio/Data Corp., Hatboro, PA.

Procedure

1. Collect 4.5 ml patient's blood in 0.5 ml anticoagulant solution. Centrifuge at high speed for 10 minutes and remove plasma within 1 hour. Refrigerate plasma until ready to use.
2. Place 4 tubes in 37°C water bath and add 0.2 ml control plasma to 2 tubes, and 0.2 ml patient's plasma to the other 2. Allow to warm 3 minutes.

3. Blow 0.1 ml thrombin solution, which has been kept in a plastic tube at room temperature, into one of the control pair and determine the clotting time. If the time is not between 10 and 15 seconds, adjust the thrombin concentration.
4. Test the other control sample and both of the patient's samples.
5. The same procedure may be followed, using the regular thrombin-calcium solution. With this reagent, the clot will be more opaque and the control time shorter if an equal concentration of thrombin is used.
6. If the patient's average clotting time exceeds the average control time by a factor of 1.3 with either reagent, the test should be repeated on a 1:1 mixture of the patient's and control plasmas.
7. The special thrombin-calcium solution, (No. 6) should be used for testing heparinized plasma.

Interpretation

If the patient's thrombin time is significantly longer than the control, this suggests either a marked deficiency of factor I (fibrinogen), a structural abnormality in the fibrinogen molecules, or the presence of inhibitors of the thrombin-fibrinogen reaction. If the 1:1 mixture of the patient, and control plasmas gives a clotting time approximating that of the control plasma, deficiency or structural abnormality of the fibrinogen is the likely diagnosis. If the clotting time of the mixture is nearer that of the patient's plasma, this suggests the presence in the patient's plasma of inhibitor activity. If the disparity between the thrombin times of the patient and the control is much more apparent with the pure thrombin solution than with the thrombin-calcium solution, this definitely suggests a structural abnormality in the fibrinogen molecules. If thrombin times are normal with both thrombin and thrombin-calcium reagents but the clots are all of poor quality, this suggests a deficiency of factor XIII.

The thrombin-calcium clotting time can be used in monitoring heparin therapy. If it is to be used in this way, it is recommended that a heparin control curve be prepared. (See page 129 for directions for preparing heparin concentrations for testing.)

FIBRINOGEN ASSAYS

General Principles

Because of the lack of sensitivity of the standard thrombin time to changes in fibrinogen levels, the test has been altered to improve its value in quantitatively measuring fibrinogen by diluting the plasma sample (1:10) and adding an excess of thrombin (100 U/ml) to overcome the influence of inhibitors (Clauss method). This method is satisfactory for use in a bleeding emergency and in the evaluation of patients with DIC because it can be completed quickly and can be done by minimally trained personnel.

The classic assay procedure, on the contrary, is tedious and time-consuming. The concentration of clottable fibrinogen is determined by adding thrombin or calcium chloride to plasma, washing the clot, and determining the weight or its protein content by the biuret or Folin-Ciocalteu method. Falsely low values may be obtained when an excess of antithrombin activity is present and when there is active fibrinolysis. When time is not a factor, however, this procedure gives a reliable measurement of fibrinogen and may be useful in checking the accuracy of the more rapid method.

Immunologic quantitative methods are available but require 24 hours for completion.

As mentioned in Chapter 3, one of the semiautomated instruments (Bio/Data Coagulation Profiler) that is used for performing clotting end-point tests results in a graphic display of the coagulation process called a thrombokinetogram. The maximum change in optical density (V max) that appears on the thrombokinetogram patterns of APTT, PT, or TT tests can give semiquantitative information about the level of fibrinogen, since the amplitude varies directly with the quantity of fibrinogen (Figure 9-1). An absolute value can be calculated by comparing the V max of a thrombin-time pattern of a patient's plasma to that of an assayed reference plasma; this is referred to as a thrombokinetic fibrinogen assay. The automated Dupont ACA fibrinogen assay is based on changes in optical density after the addition of thrombin.

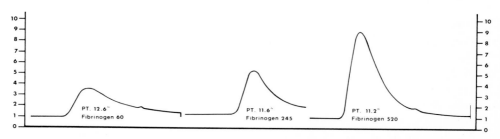

Figure 9-1.   Thrombokinetograms of prothrombin time tests on plasma samples with variable fibrinogen levels (mg/100 ml).

In some dysfibrinogenemias, thrombin times may be prolonged and a fibrinogen assay by the Clauss method may underestimate the level of fibrinogen. Normal results may be found by the thrombokinetic, gravimetric, nephelometric, or immunologic methods because they are not dependent on the rate of fibrin formation.

Careful quantitative observation of the clot during retraction gives valuable information about the fibrinogen content of blood. The more fibrinogen that is present, the larger will be the fibrin web, and the better able to retain red blood cells in the meshes. When fibrinogen is decreased, either in absolute terms or relative to the red cell mass, red cell fallout from the clot is increased. In polycythemia, when the red cell mass is high and the plasma volume proportionally low, there is rarely enough fibrinogen to retain all of the red cells in the clot, and the red cell fallout may be so great as to suggest fibrinolysis. Euglobulin clot lysis in such cases is usually normal, however, thus ruling out lysis as a significant causal mechanism.

Clauss Method

Reagents

1. Sodium citrate (3.8%), sodium oxalate (0.1 *M*), or acid-citrate solution.
2. Barbital-buffered saline.
3. Thrombin solution. A stock solution may be made by adding 10 ml 50% glycerol in barbital-buffered saline to a vial containing 1000 U bovine topical thrombin (Parke-Davis, Detroit, MI), giving a concentration of 100 U/ml.

4. Freshly prepared commercial standard plasma of known fibrinogen concentration.
5. 2-cycle log-log graph paper.
6. Fibrinogen determination kits are available from Dade and Ortho, which contain thrombin reagent, fibrinogen standard, and barbital-buffered saline.
7. A fibrometer is useful in performing this test.

Procedure

1. Blood may be collected by syringe or Vacutainer, combining 4.5 ml blood with 0.5 ml anticoagulant.
2. Centrifuge the blood for 10 minutes at 3000 rpm and remove plasma.
3. Using barbital-buffered saline, prepare 1:5, 1:15, and 1:40 dilutions of the standard plasma of known fibrinogen concentration.
4. Determine the clotting time of each dilution in duplicate by incubating 0.2 ml diluted plasma in the 37°C water bath for 3 minutes before forcibly blowing in 0.1 ml thrombin solution that has been kept at room temperature.
5. Average the clotting time for each dilution and plot the points on the 2-cycle log-log graph paper. The clotting times should be plotted on the ordinate and the fibrinogen concentration on the abscissa. The graph paper furnished with Dade Fibrinogen Determination Set has lines conveniently drawn for plotting each dilution of the particular fibrinogen standard furnished with the kit.
6. Dilute the patient's sample 1:10 with barbital-buffered saline and test in duplicate as was done with the dilutions of the standard plasma. Very high levels may require the testing of a 1:20 dilution and very low values the testing of 1:5 or 1:2 dilutions.
7. Read the results from the calibration curve and report in mg/100 ml, making the necessary calculations if plasma dilutions other than 1:10 are tested. If a 1:5 dilution is used, divide the result by 2; if a 1:20 is used, multiply by 2.
8. Both normal and abnormal fibrinogen controls may be tested in the same way as the patient's sample, since such plasmas are manufactured to have fibrinogen levels within a stated range.

Normal Values: 170 mg/100 ml to 410 mg/100 ml, with a mean value of 290 mg/100 ml.

Reference

Clauss A: Gerinnungsphysiologische Schneliomethode zur Bestimmung des Fibrinogens. Acta Haemat 17:237, 1957.

Folin-Ciocalteu Method
Reagents

1. Dry potassium oxalate or EDTA.
2. Calcium chloride solution (0.1 *M*).
3. Sodium hydroxide (10%).

4. Sodium carbonate (30%).
5. Phenol reagent (Folin-Ciocalteu). Into a 2000-ml Florence flask place:
       100 mg sodium tungstate
        25 mg sodium molybdate
       700 ml distilled water
        50 ml 85% phosphoric acid
       100 ml concentrated hydrochloric acid
    Reflux gently for 10 hours. Add 150 g lithium sulfate, 50 ml distilled water, and a few drops of bromine. Remove the excess bromine by boiling. Cool and dilute to 1000 ml with distilled water. If the reagent develops a green color, it is again treated with bromine and boiled. This reagent is also available commercially.
6. Tyrosine standard stock solution is prepared by dissolving 200 mg pure tyrosine in 1000 ml 0.1 N hydrochloric acid: 1 ml = 0.2 mg tyrosine.

Procedure

1. Collect blood with either dry potassium oxalate or EDTA. Dilute 1.0 ml plasma with 25 ml distilled water in a beaker and add 2 ml 0.1 M calcium chloride solution.
2. After 30 minutes, remove the voluminous clot that has formed by wrapping it onto a stirring rod. Thoroughly wash the clot in distilled water, remove it from the glass rod, and put it into a glass test tube.
3. Digest the clot by covering it with 0.5 ml 10% sodium hydroxide and heating in a boiling water bath for 10 minutes. (More accurate results are obtained if the tube is placed in a refrigerator at 4°C for 10 hours before the digestion in the boiling water bath.)
4. Dilute the alkaline solution with distilled water in a volumetric flask to 25 ml. Centrifuge a portion of the solution to remove the suspended calcium oxalate. Transfer 5 ml of the centrifuged solution to a 15 × 250 mm test tube.
5. Add 4.5 ml distilled water, 0.5 ml phenol reagent, and 3 ml 20% sodium carbonate solution. Mix by inversion and allow to stand 30 minutes for maximum color development.
6. Measure the color intensity in a Coleman Junior Spectrophotometer at 560 mμ. The value obtained is read directly in terms of tyrosine or fibrinogen from a curve.
7. The curve is prepared by diluting stock tyrosine solution and adding reagents to develop color, as in the test.

Stock tyrosine solution (ml)	0.1	0.2	0.3	0.4	0.5
Distilled water (ml)	9.5	9.5	9.5	9.5	9.5
Phenol reagent (ml)	05.	0.5	0.5	0.5	0.5
20% Na_2CO_2 (ml)	3.0	3.0	3.0	3.0	3.0
Tyrosine concentration (mg)	0.02	0.04	0.06	0.08	0.1

From the values obtained on reading the color intensities of the standards, construct a curve on semilogarithmic graph paper. The calculation is:

$$\text{mg tyrosine in sample} \times \frac{10}{9} \times 5 \times 10.7 \times 100 = \text{mg fibrinogen/100 ml plasma}$$

Normal Value: 250 to 400 mg/100 ml plasma

Reference

Quick AJ: Hemorrhagic Diseases and Thrombosis, 2nd Ed. Philadelphia, Lea & Febiger, 1966, p. 410.

Radial Immunodiffusion

The M-Partigen Fibrinogen Kit available from Calbiochem-Behring, LaJolla, CA may be used. The precision is largely a function of technique. This method may overestimate the level of clottable fibrinogen, especially when immunologically reactive FDP are present.

Normal Values: 200 to 450 mg/100 ml.

Thrombokinetic Fibrinogen Assay

The quantitative fibrinogen kit available from Bio/Data Corp., Hatboro, PA may be used with the Bio/Data Coagulation Profiler. The results are compared by dividing the product of the fibrinogen value of a calibrated reference sample and the V max of the patient's sample by the V max of the reference sample.

Normal Value: 200 to 400 mg/100 ml plasma.

QUALITATIVE TEST FOR FIBRIN STABILIZING FACTOR
(Clot Stability in 5 Molar Urea)

General Principles

Since clots formed in the absence of activated factor XIII lack stability and have been found to be soluble in concentrated urea and weak acid solutions, it is possible to test for gross deficiencies of factor XIII with the urea or monochloroacetic acid stability test. The test is very gross and is only positive when levels of factor XIII are below 1% or 2%. Calcium is required for the activation of factor XIII by thrombin; when factor XIII is lacking, there is little difference in the appearance of a clot formed with or without calcium chloride.

Technique

Reagents

1. Sodium citrate solution (3.8%).
2. Calcium chloride (0.025 *M*).
3. Urea solution, 5 *M* (dissolve 30 g urea in 100 ml distilled water). Alternatively, 1% monochloroacetic acid can be used.

Procedure

1. Collect 4.5 ml blood into 0.5 ml sodium citrate solution. Centrifuge and separate plasma.
2. Place 0.1 ml plasma in a tube in the 37°C water bath and add 0.1 ml calcium chloride solution. Allow to clot and to stand in the water bath for 30 minutes.
3. Tap the clot loose and add 3 ml urea solution or 1 ml of monochloroacetic acid solution. Allow the tube to stand at room temperature; inspect at intervals for the disappearance of the clot.

Normal Values: Normal clots always survive over 24 hours. A level of 1 to 2% of factor XIII will produce a clot that is insoluble in a 5 *M* urea solution or 1% monochloroacetic acid.

Reference

Losowsby MA, Hall R, and Goldie W: Congenital deficiency of fibrin stabilizing factor. Lancet 2:156, 1965.

CHAPTER *10*

Evaluation of Fibrinolysis

CLOT LYSIS TESTS

General Principles

The optimal temperature for clot lysis is body temperature or 37° C. Only when lytic activity is really excessive is it possible to demonstrate the destruction of a clot in a tube of blood that is taped to the wall or bed, as was the suggested procedure when acceleration of this mechanism was first recognized. Especially when activity is minimal, it is important to transfer the whole blood immediately to a 37° C water bath and there watch for clotting and lysis.

Plasmin is inactivated rapidly in shed blood when it is in contact with glass and when platelets and calcium are present, so little, if any, fibrinolytic activity remains in serum. Citrated plasma shows the greatest amount of sensitivity in lytic tests, and clots formed with thrombin alone are much more susceptible to lysis than those formed with calcium chloride, because calcium is required for the activation of factor XIII which strengthens the clot. For these reasons, the most sensitive tests for lysis call for the collection of blood with citrate, the rapid separation and testing of plasma, and the use of thrombin to form the clot.

If fibrinogen is absent or significantly decreased, it is impossible to test for fibrinolysis unless additional fibrinogen is supplied by normal plasma or commercial material. Therefore, a quantitative or semiquantitative determination of fibrinogen should be an essential part of fibrinolytic studies. The best test systems are the diluted whole-blood clot lysis or the euglobulin clot lysis tests. If fibrinogen is found to be absent or significantly decreased, normal plasma or commercial fibrinogen must be added to the patient's plasma before testing. Findings may include hypofibrinogenemia alone, increased fibrinolytic activity alone, or a combination of the two.

Because of the effectiveness of the inhibitor system and the slow rate at which fibrinolysis normally occurs, it is not easy to demonstrate it in the laboratory. Unless some artificial method is used to dilute or remove inhibitors, determination of the presence of pathologic fibrinolytic activity may require at least 24 hours. The diluted whole-blood clot lysis test takes advantage of dilution to decrease inhibitor activity and also utilizes an initial 30-minute period of refrigeration, which tends to further

169

inactivate inhibitors and slow the loss of fibrinolytic activity. Since this test is performed on nonanticoagulated blood, it must be initiated immediately after the venipuncture is done, and therefore, is a practical procedure only when this is possible.

The euglobulin lysis time test measures the rate of lysis of a clot artificially prepared from the euglobulin proteins of plasma. These proteins, which precipitate when plasma is diluted and slightly acidified, include plasminogen activator, fibrinogen, and plasminogen, but not antiplasmins and antiplasminogen activator. Only about 50 % of the original fibrinogen is usually present in the precipitate, which is resuspended in buffered saline and clotted with thrombin. Lysis of such a euglobulin clot normally occurs more rapidly than lysis of a whole-blood or plasma clot. The test is considered normal if the clot requires more than 1½ hours to lyse, but if proteolysis is especially active, the clots may be lysed within 15 minutes. The test measures primarily uninhibited activator activity. It may be somewhat more sensitive than the diluted whole-blood clot lysis test and it can be easily done on patients receiving heparin, since the heparin is removed during the precipitation process. Also, it can be done on a plasma sample and does not require that the technologist be ready to proceed with testing immediately after the blood is drawn as is required with the diluted whole-blood clot lysis test.

The following set of rules may be useful in carrying out tests to demonstrate the lysis of fibrin so that they will give a maximum of information.

1. Since fibrinolytic activity can be influenced by irritation of the vein, venous stasis, anxiety, and medications, the blood should be drawn carefully, without stasis, in a clean, dry syringe.
2. Normally, fibrinolytic activity is increased in samples drawn after a specified period of venous stasis produced by an occlusive blood pressure cuff. The comparison of samples drawn before and after occlusion is useful in the evaluation of activator release.
3. Citrate is the best anticoagulant for plasma tests. Blood so collected should be processed within 30 minutes, the plasma being kept in an ice bath until ready for use.
4. Thrombin should be used to clot plasma or blood, the optimal amount being about 10 units per ml.
5. For complete evaluation of fibrinolysis, knowing the fibrinogen level is essential because it affects the structure and size of the clot. If plasma fibrinogen is significantly decreased, it is impossible to evaluate fibrinolysis without adding commercial fibrinogen or normal plasma to the patient's blood.
6. Dilution of blood or plasma decreases inhibitor activity.
7. Precipitation of plasma by dilution and acidification removes inhibitor activity.
8. Refrigeration slows the loss of fibrinolytic activity.

Many elements must be considered in selecting tests for the evaluation of fibrinolytic activity in a patient. All the regularly used procedures have limitations, and it may often be necessary to do more than one test in order to fully understand the situation. In a patient described as having an α-2-antiplasmin deficiency, the whole-blood clot lysis and dilute-plasma clot lysis times were abnormally short, but the euglobulin clot

TABLE 10-1.   Comparison of Clot Lysis Tests

Test	Measures	Sensitivity	Test Required (hours)
Whole blood clot lysis	Activator Plasminogen (plasmin) Fibrinogen Inhibitors	+/−	24
Diluted whole blood clot lysis	Activator Plasminogen (plasmin) Fibrinogen Inhibitors (decreased)	++	2–12
Euglobulin clot lysis	Activator Plasminogen (plasmin) Fibrinogen (decreased) Inhibitors (eliminated)	++ or +++	2

lysis time was normal because, in the latter test, inhibitors are eliminated. Visible lysis of fibrin is the end point for all tests. Table 10-1 gives a comparative evaluation of the most useful procedures.

References

Bjorkman SE, (ed): Hereditary Coagulation Disorders—Fibrinolysis. Copenhagen, Munksgaard, 1965, p. 70.

Miles LA, et al: A bleeding disorder due to a deficiency of α 2 antiplasmin. Blood 59:1246, 1982.

Sirridge MS, Bowman AB, and Garber PE: Fibrinolysis and changes in fibrinogen in multiple myeloma. Arch Intern Med 101:630, 1958.

von Kaulla KN: Chemistry of Thrombolysis, Human Fibrinolytic Enzymes. Springfield, Charles C Thomas, 1963.

Whole-Blood Clot Lysis

Procedure

1. Place 2 ml whole blood in each of 3 glass test tubes and place immediately in 37°C water bath.
2. Observe for formation of the clot; leave 2 tubes in the water bath and place one in the refrigerator.
3. Observe at intervals for 24 hours for degeneration or disappearance of the clot.

Interpretation

Normally, the clot will remain intact at least 48 hours. If the clot dissolves within 24 hours, lysis is considered to be increased. If the clot appears to have disappeared, pour the contents of one tube on a piece of filter paper to be certain no clot is present. If fibrinogen is present in normal amounts, the refrigerated specimen should retain a firm clot, and thus serves as a control. If clot formation seems defective and there is no clot or only a small, friable clot in the refrigerated tube, this indicates a deficiency of fibrinogen rather than increased lysis (Figure 10-1).

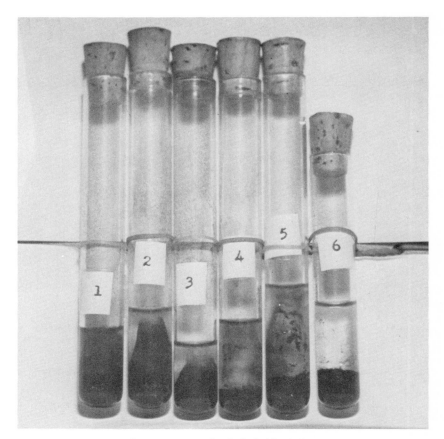

Figure 10-1. Lysis of whole blood clots.

Diluted Whole-Blood Clot Lysis

Reagents

1. Phosphate buffer (pH 7.4). Dissolve 9.47 g Na_2HPO in 1.0 L of distilled water. To this add 3.02 g KH_2PO_4 dissolved in 250 ml distilled water. Sterilize the buffer by heat method and keep in the refrigerator.
2. Barbital-buffered saline.
3. Thrombin solution. To a vial containing 1000 units of bovine topical thrombin add 10 ml of 50% glycerol in barbital-buffered saline. Store this in the freezer until ready for use. Then further dilute this stock solution 1 : 2 with barbital-buffered saline to give a solution containing 50 U/ml.

Procedure

1. Into each of 3 plain glass tubes (in an ice bath) place 1.70 ml phosphate buffer and 0.1 ml thrombin solution, the latter being added just before the test is started.

2. Obtain 1.0 ml blood by venipuncuture and place this in a tube. Immediately add 0.2 ml to each of the tubes containing buffer and thrombin, tilting gently once.
3. Place the tubes in a refrigerator for one-half hour to inactivate the inhibitors.
4. Remove 2 of the tubes to a 37°C water bath. After 10 minutes, carefully rotate the tubes between the palms of the hands to loosen the retracting clots.
5. Retraction proceeds uniformly until the clots have retracted to about one tenth of their original size and are floating in the buffer.
6. Lysis is first noted as a shagginess, followed by complete disappearance of the clots.
7. The tube that is left in the refrigerator serves as a control. The presence of a clot in this tube is evidence of the presence of fibrinogen in the blood. Lysis does not occur at refrigerator temperature. This clot will lyse when placed in the 37°C water bath, however, even if kept in the refrigerator for 24 hours.

Normal Values: 2 to 12 hours (for blood drawn in the morning, the time is usually longer, but frequently is less than 6 hours in the afternoon. The mean in 40 patients was 5½ hours).

References

Fearnley GR: Fibrinolysis. Baltimore, Williams & Wilkins, 1965.
Fearnley GR: Spontaneous fibrinolysis. Am J Cardiol 6:371, 1960.
Fearnley GR, Balmforth GR, and Fearnley E: Evidence of a diurnal fibrinolytic rhythm with a simple method of measuring natural fibrinolysis. Clin Sci 16:645, 1957.

Euglobulin Lysis Time

Reagents

1. Sodium citrate solution (3.8%).
2. Acetic acid, 1% (W/V). Dilute 1.0 ml concentrated acetic acid to 100 ml with distilled water.
3. Cold distilled water.
4. Barbital-buffered saline.
5. Thrombin solution. To a vial containing 1000 units bovine topical thrombin add 10 ml 50% glycerol in a barbital-buffered saline. Store this in the freezer until ready for use. Then further dilute this stock solution 1:2 with barbital-buffered saline to give a solution containing 50 U/ml.
6. Abnormal fibrinolysis control (Dade, Miami, FL). Reconstitute one vial plasminogen activator (streptokinase) with 1.0 ml distilled water and pour the reconstituted solution into an unreconstituted vial of plasmin control.

Procedure

1. Draw 4.5 ml blood from the patient and add it to 0.5 ml sodium citrate solution, with minimal venous stasis. In cases of thromboembolic disease

in which decreased fibrinolytic activity is suspected, a second sample should be drawn after a blood pressure cuff has been placed on the other arm above a venipuncture site and maintained at 90 mm Hg for 5 minutes.

2. Centrifuge tubes rapidly in a refrigerated centrifuge, if available, and separate the plasma immediately. The plasma should be kept in an ice bath and tested within 30 minutes.

3. Add 0.5 ml of each plasma sample to 6 ml cold distilled water in a large test tube. Add 0.5 ml abnormal fibrinolysis control to another tube of 6 ml cold distilled water.

4. Add 0.1 ml 1% acetic acid to each. This should bring the pH to approximately 5.9 and produce a white precipitate.

5. Allow the mixtures to stand at 5°C for 10 minutes and then centrifuge at 3000 rpm for 10 minutes (preferably, in a refrigerated centrifuge).

6. Decant, and dry the sides of the tubes carefully with cotton tipped applicators.

7. Dissolve the precipitates in 0.35 ml barbital-buffered saline. (Use of a glass rod is necessary to aid in dissolving.)

8. Add 0.025 ml thrombin solution to each tube. Mix well and watch for clotting, which should be immediate.

9. Incubate at 37°C and check every 10 minutes for lysis.

10. If the fibrinogen level is 60 to 80 mg%, it will be necessary to repeat the test on a 1:1 mixture of patient's and normal plasma.

Interpretation

A normal euglobulin lysis time is greater than 90 minutes and the abnormal control should lyse within 30 minutes. This is a crude procedure and considerable variation in lysis time may be observed. The time can be artificially shortened by prolonged use of the tourniquet and by rubbing the vein vigorously or pumping the arm, all of which tend to release plasminogen activator. Since platelets prolong the lysis time by their antiplasmin activities, platelet-poor plasma should be used. The lower the pH of the plasma–acid mixture, the longer the lysis time. Maximal lysis is obtained by precipitating euglobulins at pH 6.2, with increasing prolongation as the pH approaches 5.3. (Euglobulin precipitated at pH 5.3 will not lyse for 10 to 24 hours.) The time will be shortened by a lack of fibrin substrate and bacterial contamination of reagents.

Normally, the lysis time of the sample drawn after venous occlusion should be considerably shorter than that of the initial sample. If shortening does not occur, this is indicative of decreased plasminogen activator release.

References

Blix S: Studies on the fibrinolytic system in the euglobulin fraction of human plasma. Scand J Clin Lab Invest *13* (Suppl 58):3, 1961.
Bowie EJW, et al: Mayo Clinic Laboratory Manual of Hemostasis. Philadelphia, W.B. Saunders, 1971.

TESTS FOR SOLUBLE MONOMER COMPLEXES (SFMC)
General Principles

In on-going, slow evolution of thrombin, fibrin monomers may be produced in quantities insufficient to support the formation of significant amounts of fibrin, but sufficient to polymerize with fibrinogen molecules and various fibrinogen-fibrin degradation products that are likewise being produced by this process. These may be recognized in plasma samples in the laboratory by the so-called paracoagulation reactions, such as the protamine sulfate tests, the ethanol gelation test, and detection of cryofibrinogen. These tests are nonspecific and must be performed carefully. It is often useful to do more than one test because apparently they do not detect exactly the same complexes. The protamine sulfate tests are more specific than the others, but may not be as sensitive as the ethanol gelation test. The ethanol gelation test may give false positive results when fibrinogen levels are over 400 mg%. Thus a negative test is of more diagnostic significance.

Plasma Protamine Paracoagulation (3P) Test
Reagents

1. Sodium citrate (3.8%), sodium oxalate (0.1 M), or acid-citrate solution.
2. Protamine sulfate, 1% solution (Lilly).

Procedure

1. Obtain blood from the patient and add 4.5 ml to 0.5 ml anticoagulant solution. Vacutainers can be used. If the hematocrit is significantly reduced, the proportion of anticoagulant should be increased.
2. Centrifuge the blood for 10 minutes at 3000 rpm and remove the plasma.
3. Place 1.0 ml of the plasma in a glass test tube and warm to 37°C for 3 minutes.
4. Add 0.1 ml of the 1% protamine sulfate solution. Mix by tilting and return to the 37°C water bath.
5. At 3 minutes and at 10 minutes, tilt the tube gently and return to the water bath.
6. After 15 minutes, remove the tube from the water bath and examine for visible white fibrin threads. A good source of light and a magnifying mirror are recommended.

Interpretation

Negative: no insoluble material.
Positive: varies from a fine, noncohesive precipitate, which may be difficult to see without a magnifying mirror, to a fibrin web, fibrin strands, or a soft conglomerate readily visible without magnification.

References

Kidder WR, Logan LJ, Rapaport SL, and Patch MJ: The plasma protamine paracoagulation test. Am J Clin Pathol 58:675, 1972.
Seaman AJ: The recognition of intravascular clotting: the plasma protamine paracoagulation test. Arch Intern Med 125:1016, 1970.

Serial-Dilution Protamine Sulfate Test

Reagents

1. Sodium citrate solution (3.8%).
2. Protamine sulfate, 1% solution, (Lilly).
3. Epsilon aminocaproic acid (EACA) (1.0 M solution). This is made by diluting EACA (Lederle, 250 mg/ml) 1:2 with distilled water.
4. Barbital-buffered saline.

Procedure

1. Draw blood from patient and add 4.5 ml to 0.5 sodium citrate solution.
2. Centrifuge for 10 minutes at 3000 rpm and remove the plasma from the cells.
3. To 1 ml platelet-poor plasma add 0.05 ml 1.0 M EACA.
4. Mix a fresh 1% solution of protamine sulfate with barbital-buffered saline in the following 4 dilutions: 1:5, 1:10, 1:20, and 1:40.
5. Transfer 0.2 ml of each dilution to a glass test tube.
6. Add 0.2 ml plasma to be tested to each of 4 tubes containing 0.2 ml volumes of protamine sulfate dilutions, and mix the tubes gently. The final concentrations of protamine sulfate in the mixtures are 1000, 500, 250, and 125 μg/ml.
7. Examine the tubes after 30 minutes and again after 24 hours of standing corked at room temperature.

Interpretation

1. Under these conditions, large soluble fibrin monomer complexes tend to polymerize early; whereas the polymerization reaction of smaller complexes with fibrin degradation products is delayed. A distinction can sometimes be made between these two products, therefore, by making observations at 30 minutes and at 24 hours.
2. The appearance of material in the test tubes is described as follows:
   g = gelation
   fs = fibrin strand
   fy = feathery precipitate
   The test is considered unequivocally positive if fibrin strands or gelation develops at any dilution and weakly positive if feathery precipitate formation is seen.
3. If the test is positive, additional quantitative information may be obtained by diluting the test plasma with a barbital-citrate buffer (9:1 mixture of barbital-buffered saline and 3.8% sodium citrate). Serial dilutions (1:2, 1:4, 1:8, and 1:16, and so forth) of the plasma are made with the barbital-citrate buffer, and the serial-dilution protamine sulfate test is performed on each dilution of plasma. The last plasma dilution giving a positive reaction is recorded.

Reference

Gurewich V, and Hutchinson E: Detection of intravascular coagulation by a serial-dilution protamine sulfate test. Ann Intern Med 75:895, 1971.

Ethanol Gelation Test

Reagents

1. Sodium citrate solution (3.8%).
2. Borate buffer (0.15 M, pH 8.0). The stock solution is made by mixing 0.15 M boric acid with 0.15 M sodium borate to achieve a pH of 8.0.
3. Ethanol-borate buffer. Mix 650 ml stock borate buffer with 150 ml absolute ethanol. This reagent is stable indefinitely at room temperature.

Procedure

1. Draw blood from the patient and add 4.5 ml to 0.5 ml sodium citrate solution.
2. Centrifuge for 10 minutes at 3000 rpm and remove the plasma from the cells.
3. Place 0.5 ml platelet-poor plasma in a test tube.
4. Add 0.8 ml ethanol-borate buffer and mix.
5. Leave at room temperature and read at 10-, 20-, 30-, and 60-minute intervals.

Interpretation

Definite strands or gel at 10 minutes constitutes a positive test. Any strands appearing later have doubtful significance. The appearance of a flock without a definite strand or gel at any time has doubtful significance.

Cryofibrinogen

Either citrated or oxalated plasma that has been left over from coagulation studies should be divided into two equal portions in glass tubes. One tube should be covered and left at room temperature, and the other should be placed in the refrigerator overnight. The two tubes should be compared the next day. Cryofibrinogen may appear as a heavy precipitate, a few strands, or a gel in the refrigerated specimen only. Usually, it will disappear when the plasma is warmed to 37°C. If only a small amount of plasma is available and serum from the same patient is available, an alternate procedure may be used. Both plasma and serum in tubes should be placed in a refrigerator overnight. If the plasma tube shows flocculation or gelation that is absent in the serum tube, this suggests the presence of a cryofibrinogen. Flocculation or gelation in both serum and plasma suggests the presence of a cryoglobulin.

TESTS FOR THE PRESENCE IN SERUM OF FIBRINOGEN-FIBRIN DEGRADATION PRODUCTS

General Principles

Another approach to the diagnosis of fibrinolysis is the demonstration in serum of fibrinogen-fibrin degradation products (FDP), which are produced by the proteolytic action of plasmin on fibrin or fibrinogen. Studies of fibrinogenolysis after administration of a plasminogen activator have demonstrated three stages of proteolysis of fibrinogen (Figure 1-6). A large fragment X is formed within 15 minutes (stage 1). This fragment is further degraded to smaller ones called, Y, D, and E within the next 60 minutes (Stage II). At the end of 6 hours, fragments D and E remain (stage III). These fragments vary in their immunologic and anticoagulant activity. If blood is collected carefully, with the addition of thrombin to assure complete clotting and a soybean trypsin inhibitor to prevent in vitro clot lysis, the demonstration of significant amounts of any of these degradation products in serum is diagnostic of active in vivo fibrinolysis or fibrinogenolysis. Many test systems have been recommended for the detection of FDP. These tests cannot distinguish between fibrinogen and fibrin breakdown products.

The tanned red cell hemagglutination inhibition immunoassay (TRCHII) test of Merskey has been the preferred research method because of its sensitivity: however, special requirements for proper preparation and preservation of tanned erythrocytes have prevented its general use. The Wellcome FDP Kit that is based on this method is sensitive to 0.6 to 1.25 μg/ml fibrinogen equivalent (HAI FDP). For routine clinical investigation, however, the Thrombo-Wellco slide test based on a latex reagent sensitized with anti-FDP antibodies is more useful for the detection of such products and is sensitive to concentrations of 2 μg/ml fibrinogen equivalent (Latex FDP). These methods show fairly good correlation (Figure 10-2).

The staphylococcal clumping test for FDP is based on the fact that most strains of staphylococcus aureus have present in their cell walls a factor that produces visible clumping in the presence of large fibrinogen-fibrin breakdown products and fibrin monomers. This test is much easier than the TRCHII test and seems to be of adequate sensitivity to detect significant amounts of FDP, although it is less sensitive than the TRCHII test to the smaller late-degradation products. Prolongation of clotting tests such as the thrombin time requires rather large concentrations of FDP and is much more marked when stage II products are present (X, Y, D, E), since these probably polymerize readily with fibrin monomers and delay clotting.

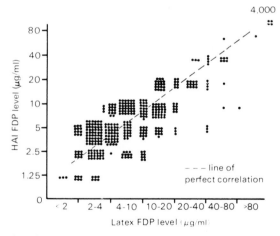

Figure 10-2. Comparison between HAI and Latex FDP levels using serum samples. (Courtesy of Wellcome Diagnostics, a division of Burroughs Wellcome Co.)

The relative sensitivity of three tests to levels and types of fibrinogen-fibrin degradation products is shown in Table 10-2. Mild to moderate increases of fibrinogen-fibrin degradation products may be found in carcinomatosis, alcoholic cirrhosis of

TABLE 10-2. Sensitivity of Tests to Levels of Various Fibrinogen-Fibrin Degradation Products

Test	Stage I (X) μg/ml	Stage II (XYDE) μg/ml	Stage III (DE) μg/ml
TRCHII	0.5-1.0	1.0-2.0	2
Staphylococcal clumping	2.5	12.5	250
Anticoagulant activity	300-600	800	1200

the liver, and during late pregnancy and parturition. In patients with eclampsia and abruptio placentae, the levels are high. Venous thrombosis and pulmonary embolism may be associated with moderate to marked increases.

References

Ellman L, et al: The Thrombo-Wellcotest as a screening test for disseminated intravascular coagulation. N Engl J Med 288:633, 1973.
Erickson C, et al: Evaluation of methods for the detection and quantitation of serum fibrin-fibrinogen degradation products. Am J Clin Pathol 58:394, 1972.
Merskey C, Lalezari P, and Johnson AJ: A rapid, simple, sensitive method for measuring fibrinolytic split products in human serum. Proc Soc Exp Biol Med 131:871, 1969.

Thrombo-Wellcotest (FDP)

Equipment and Reagents

Thrombo-Wellcotest Kit (Burroughs-Wellcome Co., Granville, NC)
1. Vacutainer collection tubes (contain soybean trypsin and thrombin).
2. Glass test slide.
3. Disposable pipettes.
4. Disposable mixing rods.
5. Latex suspension (polystyrene latex particles coated with anti-FDP globulin).
6. Positive control serum.
7. Negative control serum.
8. Glycine-saline buffer, pH 8.2.

Sample Collection

1. Obtain blood from the patient by means of a Vacutainer or use the two-syringe technique. Add 2 ml to the tube containing the soybean trypsin and thrombin and mix. The blood will clot firmly within a few seconds.
2. Rim the clot and let it stand at room temperature or 37°C for 30 minutes.
3. Centrifuge at 3000 rpm for 10 minutes. Note: if the patient is receiving heparin, the thrombin in the sample tube may be inhibited and the blood may fail to clot. If this occurs, add 2 ml of patient's heparinized blood to a plain tube containing Reptilase-R (Abbott) and mix. Blood should clot after a short incubation period at 37°C. Immediately after the sample has clotted firmly, it may be centrifuged. The clear serum obtained is suitable for assay.

Procedure

1. Place 0.75 ml glycine-saline buffer in each of 2 test tubes.
2. Using the disposable dropper provided in the kit, add 5 drops of the serum sample to one test tube. Label and mix well (approximately 1 : 5 dilutions).
3. Using the same disposable dropper, add 1 drop of the serum sample to the second tube. Label and mix well. (approximately 1 : 20 dilution).
4. Transfer 1 drop from the first tube to position 1 of the reaction slide.
5. Transfer 1 drop from the second tube to position 2 of the reaction slide.
6. Transfer 1 drop of the negative control to position 3 of the reaction slide.
7. Transfer 1 drop of the positive control to position 4 of the reaction slide.
8. Mix the latex suspension by shaking the container vigorously and add 1 drop to each position.
9. Stir each serum-latex mixture with a clean disposable mixing rod. Spread each pool of liquid until the circle is filled.
10. Rock the slide gently to and fro for a maximum of 2 minutes in front of an adequate light source.
11. Look for macroscopic agglutination.

Interpretation

1. Negative control: no agglutination.
2. Positive control: agglutination.
3. Patient's serum
    a. 1 : 5 dilution, negative agglutination: report less than 10 μg/ml FDP.
    b. 1 : 5 dilution, positive agglutination, 1 : 20 dilution, negative agglutination: report as 10 to 40 μg/ml FDP.
    c. 1 : 5 dilution, positive agglutination, 1 : 20 dilution, positive agglutination: report in excess of 40 μg/ml FDP.

Reference

Thrombo-Wellcotest, package insert. Breckenham, England, Wellcome Research Laboratories, 1974.

Staphylococcal Clumping Test

Reagents

1. EACA-thrombin solution for collecting blood samples. Add EACA solution (Sigma, 18 mg/2 drops) to a thrombin vial containing 10 NIH units thrombin (Sigma). Special Vacutainer tubes used in Thrombo-Wellcotest containing soybean trypsin and thrombin can be used.
2. Barbital-buffered saline.
3. Positive fibrinogen control. (A 1 : 10,000 dilution of a fibrinogen reference plasma will give a testing concentration of 0.2 to 0.4 μg/ml. This is the concentration we are interested in being able to detect. A commercial control having an assayed amount of fibrinogen may be used. Sigma furnishes a dried fibrinogen control containing 80 μg/vial, which is diluted initially with a Trizma albumin solution and finally with a Trizma saline buffer to give variable concentrations from 0.025 μg to 4 μg/ml for comparison with dilutions of the test serum.

4. Staphylococcal clumping factor (Sigma). Reconstitute according to directions.

Procedure

1. Collect 5 ml blood and add to EACA-thrombin solution or collect 2 ml blood in a special Thrombo-Wellcotest Vacutainer tube.
2. Mix and place tube in 37°C water bath for 2 hours. Centrifuge for 10 minutes at 3000 rpm and remove the serum with a Pasteur pipette.
3. Slide method. Mix 0.05 ml serum to be tested on a microscope slide with 0.05 ml staphylococcal bacterial suspension. Rock the mixture gently for 2 minutes at room temperature, and observe for clumping against a black background. The test slide is compared with controls consisting of 0.05 ml buffered saline and 0.05 ml bacterial suspension (negative control) and 0.05 ml diluted positive fibrinogen control and 0.05 ml bacterial suspension (positive control).
4. Test tube method. Mix 0.1 serum to be tested in a test tube with 0.05 ml staphylococcal bacterial suspension. Shake the mixture and add 0.05 ml buffered saline. Examine the tube for clumping after 30 minutes of incubation at room temperature, with the use of direct light and a black background. Read sample against controls as described in the slide method.

Note: A comparison of both slide and tube methods demonstrated that the slide method is the more sensitive technique. If a sample is positive, a clumping titer can be run by making serial dilutions of the serum and repeating the test. The titer is expressed as a reciprocal of the highest dilution of tested material giving a positive reaction. If the Sigma fibrinogen control is used, serial dilutions of serum should be compared with dilutions of the control. Calculation is made by finding the fibrinogen control that most closely matches the clumping intensity of the end point of the serum. The answer may then be expressed in fibrinogen equivalents by multiplying the reciprocal of the highest dilution of the serum giving a positive end point by the micrograms of fibrinogen in the closest matching control.

Normal Values: Positive tests with serum dilutions of 1 : 8 or greater are considered abnormal. If the Sigma fibrinogen control is used, the following interpretation is suggested:

Normal: up to 4 μg fibrinogen equivalents/ml.
Borderline: 5 to 7 μg fibrinogen equivalents/ml.
Elevated: 8 μg or more fibrinogen equivalents/ml.

MEASUREMENT OF PLASMINOGEN AND ANTIPLASMIN
General Principles

Plasminogen is the inactive precursor of plasmin and is present in circulating plasma in large amounts. Its concentration, as is that of other acute-phase reactants, is increased in conditions such as trauma, infections, and acute myocardial infarction. Levels are low in infants and in individuals with cirrhosis. In vivo, plasminogen can be activated to plasmin by a variety of mechanisms, the most important of which is the release of tissue activator from endothelial cells. Plasminogen is depleted in disseminated intravascular coagulation when secondary fibrinolysis occurs. Depletion may occur also in patients subjected to cardiopulmonary bypass. With the use of streptokinase and urokinase as thrombolytic agents, plasminogen is rapidly converted to plasmin, but the concentration returns to normal within 24 hours after the cessation of therapy. The systemic activation of plasminogen to plasmin also results in a decrease in antiplasmin, which actively neutralizes it.

Our experience in the measurement of plasminogen has been with a synthetic fluorogenic-substrate assay in which inactive plasminogen in a patient's plasma sample is activated to plasmin by incubation with streptokinase. A portion of the activated samples is then mixed with a fluorogenic synthetic substrate that has high specificity for plasmin (D-valine-leucine-lysine 5-amidoisophthalic acid dimethylester). The plasmin cleaves the fluorescent molecule and the amount of fluorescence is measured kinetically in the protopath fluorometer. Levels are determined by comparison with an assayed reference material.

Plasminogen (Synthetic Fluorogenic-Substrate Assay)

Equipment

1. Protopath fluorometer (Dade, Miami, FL).
2. Plastic test tubes 12 × 75 mm.
3. Pipettes that can measure 5.0 ml, 1.0 ml, 0.15 ml, 0.2 ml, 0.1 ml, and 10 μl.
4. 37°C heating block or water bath.
5. Vortex mixer.

Reagents

1. Protopath Plasminogen Synthetic Substrate Assay Kit. (Dade, Miami, FL).
    a. Plasminogen reference reagent. (Assay value in CTA units is recorded with the kit.) Reconstitute with 0.2 ml distilled water, restopper vial, and swirl until dissolved. Store at 2 to 8°C. Can be used for 24 hours.
    b. Streptokinase reagent. Reconstitute with 5.0 ml distilled water, restopper vial, and mix until dissolved (2000 U/ml). Store at 2 to 8°C or freeze at −20°C. Can be used for 8 hours. Since the quantity is adequate for 9 determinations, the unused material should be frozen if not used in 8 hours. It can be frozen and thawed twice.
    c. Plasminogen substrate. The lyophilized preparation of substrate, buffer, and stabilizer is packaged in disposable cuvettes (5 per package) in a foil pouch. Cuvettes must be stored at 2 to 8°C and must be used within 7 days after opening the pouch. Reconstitute each cuvette with 1.0 ml distilled water (0.8 μM/ml substrate). Stable for 4 hours at room temperature or 8 hours at 2 to 8°C after reconstitution.
2. Sodium citrate solution (3.8%).

3. Control plasma (SNP, Dade, Miami, FL). Reconstitute with 1 ml distilled water. Expected range is recorded for each lot number.

Procedure

1. Obtain blood from patient and add 4.5 ml to 0.5 ml sodium citrate solution. Vacutainers can be used.
2. Centrifuge sample for 10 minutes at 3000 rpm and remove plasma.
3. Store in a plastic tube at 2 to 8°C until tested. Sample may be stored frozen at -20°C for up to 30 days.
4. Turn on protopath fluorometer and leave sample compartment cover closed. Allow approximately 45 minutes for the instrument to reach 37.5° (± 0.2) C before use.
5. Reconstitute one vial of plasminogen reference reagent, the required number of vials of streptokinase reagent (9 tests per vial) and one vial of control plasma (SNP).
6. For each sample of be tested (plasminogen reference reagent, control plasma (SNP), and patient samples), place 0.5 ml streptokinase reagent in an appropriately labeled plastic tube.
7. Prepare activation mixtures by adding 10 μl plasminogen reference reagent, control plasma (SNP), and patient's plasma samples to each tube respectively. Mix (vortex) and incubate for 10 minutes at 37°C. When incubation is completed, samples should be tested within 4 hours if stored at room temperature and 8 hours if stored at 2 to 8°C.
8. For each test sample, reconstitute one plasminogen substrate cuvette with 1.0 ml distilled water. Do not invert cuvettes.
9. Warm cuvettes in heating block of fluorometer at least 5 minutes before adding the activated samples.
10. Check and calibrate the instrument according to instructions for its operation.
11. Add 0.1 ml plasminogen reference activation mixture to a cuvette containing prewarmed plasminogen substrate and mix by reusing the pipette tip repeatedly.
12. Place the cuvette in the sample well of the fluorometer and press READ. The display will flash on and off and the reading is taken when the display is no longer flashing. Pressing the DAMP ON may stabilize the reading. The display value should be divided by 10 to determine the level in CTA (Committee on Thrombolytic Agents) units/ml and should be within 0.2 CTA units of the value recorded with the kit for this reference sample. Variation should be ± 3 digits. It may be necessary to adjust the calibrator control to alter the rate reading for the plasminogen reference control and also for the solid reference (which is used during initial calibration of the instrument) if the variation is greater than this.
13. Test the activation mixture of the control plasma (SNP) in the same way. If the fluorometer is properly calibrated, the value for this should be within the assay range for the lot of control plasma (SNP) being used.

14. Test patient's samples in the same way. Readings must be obtained within 10 minutes after the activated sample is added to the substrate and the cuvette is placed in the sample well.
15. Determine the values by dividing the display readout results by 10 to give CTA U/ml.

Normal Range: 3.1 ± 0.7 CTA U/ml.

References
Protopath Proteolytic Enzyme Detection System. Plasminogen Synthetic Substrate Assay, Package insert. Miami, Dade, 1970.
Triplett DA, et al: Clinical Studies of the use of a fluorogenic substrate assay method for the determination of plasminogen. Thromb Haemost 42:50, 1979.

Addendum:

Plasminogen can also be measured by an alpha-caseinolytic method, a synthetic chromogenic-substrate assay (automated Dupont ACA), and radial immunodiffusion method, but we do not have personal experience with these methods.

Antiplasmin can be measured by a synthetic chromogenic-substrate assay, with which we have no experience.

Triplett DA, and Harms CS: Procedures for a Coagulations Laboratory. Chicago, ASCP, 1981.

CHAPTER *11*

Tests Useful in the Diagnosis of Hypercoagulability and Intravascular Clotting

GENERAL PRINCIPLES

No specific pattern of tests can always give definitive information about hypercoagulability and intravascular clotting because there are multiple causes for the defects, the extent and degree of severity may vary over a wide time span, and the process may be acute or chronic. As discussed in Chapter 2 (p. 47) abnormalities related to hypercoagulability can include alterations in platelet numbers and function, acceleration of coagulation reactions with or without increased levels of clotting factors, decreases in levels of normal physiologic inhibitors of clotting, and decreased fibrinolytic activity. Testing for such abnormalities can be helpful in evaluating patients in whom a tendency to thrombosis has already been demonstrated or in whom it is suspected.

Localized intravascular clotting is not likely to produce significant changes in hemostatic tests although such processes are more likely to occur in subjects who show evidence of a hypercoagulable state. With significant disseminated intravascular coagulation (DIC), however, laboratory testing reveals a wide variety of abnormalities, depending on the types, strength, and duration of the exciting stimuli and the physiologic protective mechanisms that occur.

Many tests useful in these situations have been described in previous chapters, but can be organized in the following ways to better understand their relationship to hypercoagulability and intravascular clotting.

Tests Related to Platelet Activity

All these tests have been described in Chapter 5 and include the following:

1. *Platelet counts and observation of platelet morphology.* Thrombocytosis can contribute to hypercoagulability; thrombocytopenia is frequently present in DIC.
2. *Platelet retention in glass bead columns with special Adeplat T columns.* This test can demonstrate increased adhesiveness of platelets, which is known to be related to hypercoagulability.
3. *Special aggregation tests:* spontaneous aggregation, platelet aggregation with low concentrations of aggregating agents (i.e., collagen), and the

absence of rapid platelet disaggregation with weak ADP. The usual aggregation tests are not helpful in the study of hypercoagulability, but these modifications can give important information about potential platelet hyperactivity.
4. *Measurement of platelet factor 4 and β-thromboglobulin in plasma.* An increase in either of these substances in plasma is evidence of the activation of platelets, which has caused the release reaction to take place in vivo.
5. *Circulating platelet aggregates.* Significant numbers of aggregates suggest in vivo stimulation of platelets.

Tests Related to the Speed of the Coagulation Reaction

Most of these tests have been described previously.
1. *The whole-blood clotting time, activated partial thromboplastin time (APTT), prothrombin time (PT) and thrombin time (TT).* All of these tests in some way measure the speed of clotting; however, they are designed to detect hypocoagulability rather than hypercoagulability. In most hypercoagulable states, these tests should not be prolonged. Test results vary in DIC, and the APTT, PT, and TT should be examined together. A short APTT and a slightly prolonged PT suggest early DIC. All three tests are usually prolonged in severe DIC. The TT is especially sensitive to the changes that occur in DIC and may be the only abnormal test.
2. *The thrombin generation time test (TGTT).* This test, described in this chapter, has been shown to be somewhat more useful than previously described tests in detecting accelerated coagulation.
3. *Levels of coagulation factors.* Levels of many coagulation factors may be increased, but the relationship of such increases to hypercoagulability is not clear. If the levels of activated factors could be measured, such information would be much more useful. Acute DIC characteristically produces decreases in most coagulation factors. Decreased fibrinogen is the most obvious and most easily detected of these. Chronic DIC produces a much more variable picture, and some factors may even be increased. Also, in some patients with underlying diseases, coagulation factors may be either decreased or increased for other reasons.

Tests for Physiologic Clotting Inhibitors

1. *Antithrombin III (AT III).* AT III is the most important physiologic inhibitor of intrinsic pathway reactions. Minor degrees of hypercoagulability and intravascular clotting may not result in significant, measurable decreases in AT III activity, but in DIC and serious thromboembolic states, levels may be low. Levels are increased in patients receiving oral anticoagulants. Many methods have been developed for measuring AT III and two of these are described in this chapter.
2. *β-2-macroglobulin and α-1-antitrypsin.* These inhibitors can be measured by immunologic methods, but such measurements do not appear to be of much significance in the evaluation of hypercoagulable states.

Tests Related to Clot Lysis (Chapter 10)

1. *Euglobulin clot lysis.* Decreased fibrinolytic activity is more difficult to demonstrate by this test than increased activity; but if clot lysis time is significantly increased, it could be considered a contributory factor in thrombotic states. Rarely can increased rates of clot lysis be demonstrated during active DIC except in instances in which there is concomitant liver disease. Often, decreased fibrinolytic activity is evident after an episode of DIC. Localized increased fibrinolysis may be related to bleeding after prostatectomy, but usually this is not reflected in systemic tests.

2. *Euglobulin clot lysis after venous activation.* This test can give information about the release of plasminogen activator from venous endothelium. This is necessary for the physiologic resolution of intravascular thrombi. When lysis time is not decreased after venous occlusion, this is an indication that activator activity is decreased.

3. *Levels of plasminogen and antiplasmin.* Since the conversion of plasminogen to plasmin is the normal response to intravascular clotting, the measurement of plasminogen levels may be useful in evaluating thromboembolic events. Decreased plasminogen levels may be associated with hypercoagulability, but may also reflect recent utilization as in DIC, without time for resynthesis. When there is systemic formation of plasmin, it is rapidly inactivated by antiplasmin, which may be reduced in amount.

Tests for Soluble Fibrin Monomer Complexes (SFMC) in Plasma and Fibrinogen-Fibrin Degradation Products (FDP) in Serum (Chapter 10)

1. *Tests for SFMC.* This group of tests detects the presence in plasma of soluble complexes that are formed from fibrinogen, fibrin monomers, and early degradation products of fibrinogen or fibrin. Their presence is evidence of on-going intravascular coagulation. SFMC are recognized in plasma samples by paracoagulation reactions such as the plasma protamine paracoagulation (3P) tests, the ethanol gelation test, and the detection of cryofibrinogen.

2. The presence of significant amounts of FDP in serum is good evidence that fibrinolysis or fibrinogenolysis has occurred in vivo. Normal results do not rule out these processes because such products may be rapidly cleared from the circulation. Low levels are found in a significant number of hospitalized patients. The highest levels are seen in acute DIC.

3. A related test is that for fibrinopeptide A in plasma, since this peptide is split off from fibrinogen by the action of thrombin. It can be measured by the use of an RIA kit (Mallinkrodt Inc., St. Louis, MO).

In a research study we are conducting in our laboratory, the following group of tests are included in an effort to detect hypercoagulability.

1. Platelet count.
2. Platelet aggregation with dilute collagen.
3. Thrombin generation time test (TGTT).
4. Platelet retention in Adeplat T columns to detect increased adhesiveness.
5. Serum antithrombin III activity.

In suspected DIC, the following tests are recommended for initial screening.
1. Platelet count.
2. Fibrinogen concentration.
3. APTT, PT, and TT (PT may be the most useful).
4. 3P test for SFMC.
5. Test for FDP.

THROMBIN GENERATION TIME TEST (TGTT)

This test measures the speed of the reactions of the intrinsic pathway by recalcification of plasma when there is minimal platelet activity and surface activation. It is reproducible in normal subjects; and a decreased time suggests hypercoagulability.

Equipment and Reagents

1. Sodium citrate solution (3.8%), or silicone-coated Vacutainer tubes containing 3.8% sodium citrate.
2. Glass test tubes 13 × 100 mm. (Rinse in distilled water and dry.)
3. Calcium chloride solution (0.5 M).
4. Stopwatch.

Procedure

1. Obtain blood from the patient by means of the described siliconized Vacutainer or by use of the two-syringe technique. If a syringe is used, add 4.5 ml blood to a plastic tube containing 0.5 ml sodium citrate solution.
2. Mix and centrifuge immediately for exactly 10 minutes at 3000 rpm.
3. Place a prerinsed glass test tube in 37°C water bath.
4. Pipette 1.0 ml plasma from the upper third of the plasma phase of the centrifuged sample and place it in the test tube. Do not allow plasma to run down the side of the tube.
5. Incubate at 37°C for 1 minute.
6. Carefully blow 0.1 ml calcium chloride solution into the plasma, starting the stopwatch simultaneously.
7. After 8 minutes, remove the tube from the water bath and examine for a visible clot.
8. If no clot is seen return tube to the water bath and repeat the procedure at 2-minute intervals thereafter until a clot is formed. Record this as the thrombin generation time.

Normal Range: 15 to 28 minutes.

Reference

von Kaulla KN, and von Kaulla E: Thrombin generation in normal subjects and cardiac patients. Circ Res 14:436, 1964.

ANTITHROMBIN III (AT III)

AT III Activity Clotting Assay (Serum)

To measure antithrombin III activity, a specific concentration of thrombin is added to diluted serum and the mixture is incubated. After a defined period of time, an aliquot of the mixture is withdrawn and added to a prewarmed fibrinogen solution. The resulting clotting time of the fibrinogen is a measure of the active thrombin remaining after it has been exposed to and partially neutralized by antithrombin III contained in serum. This result is compared to the clotting times of dilutions of pooled normal serum when tested with the same concentration of thrombin. Polybrene is used in the diluent to neutralize any heparin that might be present.

Equipment and Reagents

1. Fibrometer.
2. Thrombin stock solution (200 U/ml). To a 1000-unit vial of bovine topical thrombin (Parke-Davis) add 5 ml 50% solution of glycerol and barbital-buffered saline. This may be stored at $-20°C$.
3. Thrombin working solution (25 U/ml). Using a plastic pipette and test tube, dilute the stock thrombin solution 1:8 in barbital-buffered saline. Place test tube in an ice bath until ready to use.
4. Bovine-fibrinogen stock solution (1%). Dissolve dried fibrinogen without stirring in barbital-buffered saline to yield a 1% solution (room temperature). Add 1 mg $BaSO_4$ per ml of fibrinogen solution and stir the solution for 3 minutes. Centrifuge the solution 10 minutes at 3000 rpm and freeze the supernate in aliquots. Thaw one lot at 37°C immediately before use.
5. Working fibrinogen solution (0.25%). Dilute the 1% stock fibrinogen solution 1:4 in barbital-buffered saline.
6. Polybrene stock solution (10 mg/ml). Dissolve 1 g polybrene in 100 ml normal saline. Store in aliquots at $-20°C$.
7. Polybrene working solution (.005 mg/ml). Dilute the polybrene stock solution 1:10 in normal saline. Add 0.5 ml of this 1:10 dilution to 99.5 ml normal saline. Store at 4°C.
8. Normal serum pool (reference). Obtain blood from at least 10 normal donors by means of clean venipunctures, using the two-syringe technique or dry Vacutainers. If syringes are used, place the blood into glass test tubes. Keep the tubes at room temperature for approximately 2 hours. With wooden applicator sticks, loosen the clots gently from the walls of the tubes and centrifuge the tubes for 10 minutes at 3000 rpm. Separate the serum from the clots. Pool and store in aliquots at $-20°C$ until ready to use.

Procedure

1. Obtain blood from the patient in the same manner as described previously for obtaining the serum pool. With delayed clotting, the 2-hour time period should be extended until complete clotting has occurred.
2. Make test dilutions of the normal serum pool as shown in Table 11-1.
3. Pipette 0.2 ml fibrinogen working solution into fibrometer reaction cups.
4. Place 0.4 ml of the first normal serum pool dilution in a 12 × 75 ml test tube in the 37°C water bath and incubate for 1 minute.
5. With a plastic pipette, add 0.1 ml thrombin working solution to the sample, mix, and incubate for exactly 6 minutes.

TABLE 11-1.   Preparation of Test Dilutions of Normal Serum Pool for Construction of Curve for Measurement of AT III Activity

Tube	1	2	3	4	5
Dilution	1:4	1:5	1:7	1:10	1:20
% of AT III	125%	100%	75%	50%	25%
Polybrene working solution	1.5	1.6	1.7	1.8	1.9
Serum	0.5	0.4	0.3	0.2	0.1

6. At the end of the 6-minute incubation period, blow 0.1 ml of the incubation mixture into the fibrometer reaction cup containing the fibrinogen working solution and start the timer.
7. Repeat steps 3, 4, 5, and 6 for each of the 4 remaining normal serum pool dilutions. Perform duplicate determinations on each dilution. It is possible to start the incubation of successive dilutions at 1-minute intervals, thus utilizing the 6-minute incubation period necessary for each tube.
8. Calculate the average clotting time of each dilution. Plot the results on semilog graph paper with the percentages on the abscissa and the clotting times in seconds on the ordinate (logarithmic scale). Draw the "best fit" straight line through these points. This is the normal reference activity curve.
9. Repeat steps 3 through 6, substituting a 1:5 dilution of the patient's serum for the dilutions of the normal serum pool.
10. Read the percentage of activity directly from the normal reference curve after finding the point where the clotting time obtained with the 1:5 dilution of the patient's serum intercepts it.

Normal Range: 80 to 105%.

References

Bick RL, Kovacs I, and Fekete LF: A new two-stage functional assay for antithrombin III (heparin cofactor): clinical and laboratory evaluation. Thromb Res 7:745, 1976.
Grann VR, Homewood K, and Golden W: Polybrene neutralization as a rapid means of monitoring blood heparin levels. Am J Clin Pathol 58:26, 1972.
Sirridge MS, Shannon R, and Hardin WM: Effect of anticoagulant therapy on antithrombin III levels. J Am Med Wom Assoc 37:216, 1982.
von Kaulla E, and von Kaulla N: Deficiency of antithrombin III activity associated with hereditary thrombosis tendency. J Med 3:349, 1972.

Addendum

Kits are available for the measurement of antithrombin III activity in plasma. These include a clotting assay (Ortho), a synthetic chromogenic-substrate assay (Abbott, Kabi) and synthetic fluorogenic-substrate assay (Dade). An automated synthetic chromogenic-substrate assay has recently been developed (Dupont ACA). In our laboratory, we have compared results using four different activity methods (chromogenic, fluorogenic, serum, and plasma clotting methods) and have found excellent correlation. We have chosen to use the described clotting assay on serum because of our extensive experience with it and its convenience and low cost.

References

Sirridge MS, Shannon RM, and Willoughby TL: Measurement of antithrombin III in healthy subjects studied before and after taking aspirin and dipyridamole. J Am Med Wom Assoc 34:40, 1979.
Sirridge MS, Shannon R, and Hardin WM: Effect of anticoagulant therapy on antithrombin III levels. J Am Med Women Assoc 37:216, 1982.
Triplett DA, and Harms CS: Procedures for the Coagulation Laboratory. Chicago, ASCP, 1981.

AT III by Radial Immunodiffusion (Serum or Plasma)

In this method, a protein antigen in solution is applied to a cylindrical well and diffuses radially into a thin gel matrix, in which monospecific antiserum is incorporated in uniform concentrations. The antigen applied is quantitated by determining the diameter of the precipitin ring when diffusion has ceased. This indicates the combination of the applied antigen with antibody at equivalence (end point). The diameter of the precipitin ring is directly proportional to the amount of antigen applied.

Reagents

1. M-Partigen Antithrombin III Kit (Calbiochem-Behring, LaJolla, CA), which contains the following:
   a. Three antithrombin III immunodiffusion plates. These plates contain a thin layer of 2% agarose containing monospecific antihuman antithrombin III produced in rabbits. Store these at 4 to 6°C. Freezing damages the gel and extreme temperatures can cause melting. (Note expiration date).
   b. A vial of lyophilized human Protein Standard Plasma. This contains a known amount of antithrombin III, as indicated on the label, for construction of the calibration curve. Reconstitute with 0.5 ml distilled water. Stable for 7 days. (Alternate AT III QUI PLATE Kit available from Helena Lab, Beaumont, TX.)
2. Normal saline.
3. Delivery device.
4. Linear graph paper.
5. Measuring device—ruler or calibrated magnifier (Behring).
6. Plastic test tubes (12 × 75 mm).

Procedure

1. Either EDTA plasma or serum can be tested. Make a 1:2 dilution with normal saline of each sample to be tested.
2. Remove M-Partigen plate from plastic-backed aluminum foil envelope. Open plate by pressing firmly on the center of the lid with thumbs while holding lid at the periphery. Allow the plate to stand opened at room temperature for 5 minutes to allow for the evaporation of any moisture that may have condensed in the wells.

3. To construct the calibration curve, prepare 1:1, 1:2, and 1:4 dilutions of the Protein Standard Plasma with normal saline. Deliver 5 μl of the 1:1 dilution into the first well, 5 μl of the 1:2 dilution in the second, and 5 μl of the 1:4 dilution into the third well.
4. Fill wells 4 through 12 with 5 μl of the test samples.
5. Tightly close the plate and replace it in the aluminum envelope.
6. Allow it to stand in a horizontal position at room temperature for 48 hours. A preliminary reading is possible at 8 to 12 hours. Under proper refrigerated storage, precipitin rings are stable indefinitely and partly used plates may be used to test other samples if stored at 4 to 6°C and used prior to the expiration date.
7. To prepare the standard reference curve, measure the diameter (D) in millimeters of the precipitin rings of the 3 dilutions of the Protein Standard Plasma, using a ruler or calibrated magnifier. Square the diameter readings (D_2) and plot these results (ordinate) against their respective concentrations (abscissa) on linear graph paper. The concentrations must be multiplied by the dilution factor 2. Draw the best straight line that accommodates these points. This should intercept the ordinate at 11 ± 3.5 sq mm.
8. Measure the diameters of the precipitin rings for the samples tested and determine their values from the reference curve.
9. If you have a normal reference pool in your laboratory, its value in mg/100 ml can be determined and can be considered to be 100%. Samples can then be reported as percent of normal.

Normal Values: Normal human adult range is 17 to 30 mg/100 ml, with a mean of 23 mg/100 ml. (In our laboratory, the normal range is 77 to 118% of our pool, which is considered 100%.)

References

M-Partigen Antithrombin III Kit, Package Insert. LaJolla, CA, Calbiochem-Behring Corp., 1980.
Mancini G, Cardonara AO, and Heremans JF: Immunochemical quantitation of antigens by single radial immunodiffusion. Immunochemistry 2:235, 1965.
Sirridge MS, Shannon R, and Willoughby TL: Measurement of antithrombin III in healthy subjects studied before and after taking aspirin and dipyridamole. J Am Med Wom Assoc 34:40, 1979.

Addendum

Antithrombin III may also be measured immunologically by rocket immunoelectrophoresis. We have found the radial immunodiffusion method to be much simpler and as accurate and reproducible.

CHAPTER *12*

Detection of Circulating Coagulation Inhibitors

The detection of a coagulation inhibitor depends on the demonstration of a prolongation of coagulation in one or more clotting tests that cannot be corrected by the addition of normal blood or plasma. Such inhibitors are usually suspected when there is an unexpected prolongation of the activated partial thromboplastin time (APTT) in a symptomatic or asymptomatic patient. If the prolongation of clotting is not due to a circulating coagulation inhibitor, the abnormality should be corrected by as little as 10 to 20% normal plasma. Usually, however, a 1:1 mixture of normal and abnormal plasma is tested. If the clotting time of such a mixture resembles the abnormal value, an inhibitor is most likely present. The use of the APTT and PTT test systems for substitution and mixing procedures is described in Chapter 6.

Inhibitors of factors VIII, IX, XI, and XII cause prolongation of the APTT without affecting the prothrombin time (PT) or thrombin time (TT). Factor VIII inhibitors are the most important. They are highly specific, but are sometimes weak and are time- and temperature-dependent, so they may cause only slight prolongation of the APTT when fresh plasmas are tested. In patients with severe hemophilia who develop inhibitors, the APTT does not show any increased prolongation, so inhibitors must be tested for with mixing procedures. Mixtures of normal and abnormal plasmas usually give values intermediate between the two. With incubation at 37°C, however, the abnormal plasma and the mixture of normal and abnormal plasmas show significant prolongation, but the normal plasma shows little change. Freshly prepared 1:1 mixtures of incubated abnormal and normal plasmas must be tested at intervals as controls (Table 12-1). It is extremely important to determine the level of activity of a factor VIII inhibitor. This is best done by a method that measures factor VIII levels in incubated mixtures of abnormal plasma with a plasma of known factor VIII activity and allows the expression of inhibitor activity in Bethesda units.

Factor IX inhibitors are also specific but differ from factor VIII inhibitors in that they act instantly and are not temperature- or pH-dependent. Inhibitors of factors XI and XII have been described but have not been well characterized.

Factor V and factor X inhibitors cause prolongation of both the APTT and PT. Acquired factor V inhibitors usually occur transiently in the postoperative period and especially when patients have had transfusions. Inhibition of factor V is demonstrable

193

TABLE 12-1.   Use of the Partial Thromboplastin Time with Incubation of Plasma Mixtures to Demonstrate a Weak Factor VIII Anticoagulant

| | Partial Thromboplastin Time (seconds) | | | |
| | | Incubation (minutes) | | |
	Immediate	30'	60'	90'
1. Patient	120"	146"	179"	225"
2. 1:1 mixture	108"	140"	199"	225"
3. Normal	82"	84"	88"	93"
4. Fresh 1:1 mixture of 1 and 3			108"	115"

immediately when the affected patient's plasma is mixed with normal plasma, but increases progressively up to 30 minutes. Acquired factor X inhibitors may be associated with amyloidosis or viral infections. Factor VII inhibitors are rare and affect only the PT.

Antibodies to factor I have been described in afibrinogenemia. Also, some inhibitors specifically affect the conversion of fibrinogen to fibrin. They affect primarily the thrombin clotting time, but may also prolong the prothrombin time. Increased levels of globulins, as in multiple myeloma and macroglobulinemia, act in this way, as do fibrinogen-fibrin degradation products. Factor XIII inhibitors occur rarely in factor XIII-deficient and previously normal persons.

Perhaps the most interesting of the coagulation inhibitors is the lupus anticoagulant, which has become important with the increased use of the APTT as a screening test. Since abnormal bleeding rarely occurs with such inhibitors, the most important problem is their proper identification. In most instances, the APTT is moderately prolonged and the PT is normal, and the APTT is incompletely corrected in 1:1 mixtures of abnormal and normal plasmas; however, with high-titered inhibitors or a concomitant factor II deficiency, the PT is also prolonged. Since the inhibitor appears to interact with phospholipid (either provided by platelets, a partial thromboplastin reagent as in the APTT, or by the tissue-thromboplastin reagent as in the PT), there can be prolongation of the recalcification time of platelet-rich plasma, the APTT, and the PT in plasmas that contain strong inhibitors. With weaker inhibitors, the recalcification time is likely to be the most affected and the PT not at all; however, when any such inhibitor is suspected, it is useful to do the PT test using dilutions of tissue thromboplastin. If a lupus inhibitor is present, the PT done with 1:50 and 1:500 dilutions of thromboplastin will be significantly longer than that of a normal plasma tested in the same way, as shown in Table 12-2. The ratio of the result of the test on the abnormal plasma to that on the normal plasma should be <1.3.

Since one-stage assays are based on the APTT and PT tests, inhibitors may result in variable abnormalities in specific factor assays even though patient's plasmas are diluted in the assay procedures. Multiple factors often appear to be decreased.

TABLE 12-2.   Results of APTT, PT, and Tissue-Thromboplastin Inhibitor Tests of Five Patients with Lupus Anticoagulants Compared with Controls

	APTT (Sec)	APTT (Sec)	PT Pat/Cont (Sec)		
	Pat/Cont	1:1 mix	Standard	1:50 Dil.	1:500 Dil.
Patient 1	62.5/31.1	41.4	11.0/11.7	54.9/38.5	116.3/74.9
Ratio				1.4	1.6
Patient 2	60.2/38.0	44.4	11.3/10.9	48.4/33.5	113.0/72.5
Ratio				1.4	1.6
Patient 3	46.2/31.4	41.2	10.1/10.8	62.6/37.5	139.0/76.4
Ratio				1.7	1.8
Patient 4	74.3/31.7	48.3	10.6/10.9	72.6/44.1	164.9/91.0
Ratio				1.6	1.8
Patient 5	62.9/34.0	60.8	13.1/11.3	75.2/49.6	170.6/106.6
Ratio				1.5	1.6

Heparin acts with antithrombin III as an anticoagulant. All clotting tests are prolonged when significant amounts of heparin are present in the circulation. The level of therapeutic heparin activity can be determined by measuring residual thrombin activity after adding to the test plasma sample a known amount of thrombin and an excess of AT III (procedure included in this chapter).

Heparin activity can be neutralized in vivo and in vitro by protamine sulfate, and a procedure is included in this chapter for in vitro measurement of heparin activity for use in determining the amount of protamine required for in vivo neutralization.

SCREENING TEST FOR A COAGULATION INHIBITOR

Reagents

1. Sodium citrate (3.8%), sodium oxalate (0.1 M), or acid-citrate solution.
2. Activated partial thromboplastin reagent.
3. Calcium chloride solution (0.025 M).

Procedure

1. Collect blood from the patient and from a normal control, adding 4.5 ml blood to 0.5 ml anticoagulant solution. Vacutainers can be used.
2. Immediately centrifuge for 10 minutes at 3000 rpm and remove the plasma.
3. Mix the two plasmas in a series of five tubes as follows:

Tube number	1	2	3	4	5
Patient's plasma (ml)	0.0	0.1	0.2	0.5	1.0
Normal plasma (ml)	1.0	0.9	0.8	0.5	0.0

4. Perform the activated partial thromboplastin time (APTT) test on material from each tube.
5. Place the tubes in the 37°C water bath and incubate for 1 hour; repeat the APTT on material from each tube.

6. Make a fresh 1 : 1 mixture from tubes 1 and 5 and perform the APTT on this immediately. Compare the value to that obtained with tube 4 after incubation. This freshly prepared mixture is used for comparison because of possible loss of labile components during incubation of separate plasmas.
7. If there is evidence of inhibitor activity, perform both the prothrombin time (PT) test and the thrombin time (TT) test on the patient's plasma. If either is prolonged, test mixtures in the same way as was done in steps 3 and 4 with the APTT test.

Interpretation

1. Correction of the patient's abnormal APTT by normal plasma indicates that a deficient clotting factor or factors have been supplied and a coagulation deficiency is the fault.
2. If a majority of the mixtures show prolonged clotting times, a strong coagulation inhibitor is present.
3. If the initial clotting times of the mixtures are intermediate between the values for the patient and the normal control but are definitely prolonged after incubation, this suggests a weak inhibitor that progressively inactivates a clotting factor, most likely a factor VIII inhibitor.
4. If only the APTT is abnormal, a factor VIII inhibitor is most likely, but inhibitors to factors IX, XI, or XII could be the cause.
5. If the APTT and the PT are abnormal and the TT is normal, this suggests an inhibitor against factor V, factor X, or a strong lupus-type inhibitor.
6. If all three tests are abnormal, the anticoagulant activity may be due to heparin and, if so, should be able to be neutralized by protamine sulfate.
7. When fibrinogen is normal, abnormalities in the TT alone suggest the presence of fibrinogen-fibrin degradation products or hyperglobulinemia.

References

Hardisty RM, and Ingram GIC: Bleeding Disorders: Investigation and Management. Philadelphia, F.A. Davis, 1965, pp. 316-318.
Margolius R Jr, Jackson DP, and Ratnoff OD: Circulating anticoagulants: A study of 40 cases and review of the literature. Medicine 40:145, 1961.
Schleider MA, et al: A clinical study of the lupus anticoagulant. Blood 48:499, 1976.
Shapiro SS, and Hullin M: Acquired inhibitors to the blood coagulation factors. Clin Haematol 8:207, 1979.

FACTOR VIII-INHIBITOR ASSAY
(Bethesda Units)

Factor VIII inhibitors may be quantified by mixing the test plasma with a control plasma containing a known amount of factor VIII. The amount of inhibitor present can be calculated in Bethesda units by comparing the difference in factor VIII activity of a patient–control mixture and a buffer–control mixture. Since factor VIII inhibitors are time- and temperature-dependent, the mixtures are incubated at 37°C for a period of 2 hours before assaying.

Reagents

1. Sodium citrate solution (3.8%).
2. Calcium chloride solution (0.025 M).

3. Activated partial thromboplastin reagent.
4. Factor VIII-deficient substrate.
5. Barbital-buffered saline.
6. Normal plasma pool (plasma from at least five normal persons; avoid using plasma from females who are pregnant or taking oral contraceptives).

Procedure

1. Obtain blood from the patient by the two-syringe technique and add 4.5 ml blood to 0.5 ml anticoagulant. Vacutainers may be used.
2. Mix and centrifuge immediately for 10 minutes at 3000 rpm.
3. Remove plasma and store on ice. It should be tested within 2 hours.
4. Pipette 0.2 ml normal pooled plasma into each of 4 test tubes. Label one tube C (control) and 3 tubes P (patient).
5. Pipette 0.2 ml barbital-buffered saline into the C tube.
6. Dilute patient's plasma 1:5 and 1:10. (These dilutions will not be tested unless residual factor VIII activity is less than 25% when the undiluted sample is tested.)
7. Pipette 0.2 ml undiluted patient's plasma into one of the P tubes and 0.2 ml of each of the 2 dilutions into the remaining tubes and label according to dilution.
8. Mix each tube well and stopper.
9. Incubate at 37°C for 2 hours.
10. At the end of 2 hours, perform factor VIII assays on the control tube and the incubation mixture made from normal pooled plasma and undiluted patient's plasma (see page 130). Only a single dilution (1:5) of these tubes need be tested.

Precautions

1. Do not use commercial lyophilized control plasma.
2. This method is primarily for use in measuring inhibitors developed in hemophilia A, but can be used for factor IX inhibitors. If testing for a factor IX inhibitor, the 2-hour incubation period is not necessary. Mixtures can be tested immediately by performing factor IX assays.
3. Other types of inhibitors, such as the lupus type, may give erratic results with this procedure.

Calculation

1. The factor VIII activity of the control tube and patient's incubation mixture is determined from the factor VIII reference curve.
2. The residual factor VIII activity is determined by dividing the assayed factor VIII activity in the patient's incubation mixture by the assayed factor VIII activity in the control tube.

$$\text{Residual factor VIII activity (\%)} = \frac{\text{factor VIII activity (patient)}}{\text{factor VIII activity (control)}} \times 100$$

3. The residual factor VIII activity is converted to a Bethesda unit (inhibitor unit) using Table 12-3.

TABLE 12.3 Conversion of Residual Factor VIII
Activity to Bethesda Units

Residual VIII %	Bethesda Units	Residual VIII %	Bethesda Units
100.0	0.00	60.0	0.80
97.5	0.05	57.5	0.85
95.0	0.10	55.0	0.90
92.5	0.15	52.5	0.95
90.0	0.20	50.0	1.00
87.5	0.25	47.5	1.10
85.0	0.30	45.0	1.20
82.5	0.35	42.5	1.30
80.0	0.40	40.0	1.40
77.5	0.45	37.5	1.50
75.0	0.50	35.0	1.60
72.5	0.55	32.5	1.70
70.0	0.60	30.0	1.80
67.5	0.65	27.5	1.90
65.0	0.70	25.0	2.00
62.5	0.75		

4. If the residual factor VIII activity is less than 25%, the incubation mixture made of 0.2 ml normal pooled plasma and 0.2 ml 1 : 5 dilution of patient's plasma must be tested. (Higher dilution may be needed.) The inhibitor units can then be read from Table 12-3 and multiplied by the dilution factors of the diluted samples.

Normal Value: Less than 0.5 Bethesda units.

Reference

Kasper K, et al: A more uniform measurement of factor VIII inhibitors. Thromb Diath Hemorrh 34:869, 1975.

LUPUS ANTICOAGULANT
(Tissue Thromboplastin Inhibitor Test)

Patient's plasma is incubated with different dilutions of thromboplastin reagent and the clotting time is determined. The lupus anticoagulant will show inhibitory activity against diluted tissue-thromboplastin, with significant prolongation of clotting time compared with a normal control.

Reagents

1. Sodium citrate (3.8%), sodium oxalate (0.1 *M*) or acid-citrate solution.
2. Normal saline (0.9% NaCl).
3. Simplastin (General Diagnostics, Morris Plains, NJ).
4. Calcium chloride solution (0.025 *M*).
5. Normal control plasma.

Procedure

1. Collect blood by syringe or Vacutainer, combining 4.5 ml blood with 0.5 ml anticoagulant.
2. Centrifuge the blood for 10 minutes at 3000 rpm and remove plasma.
3. To 0.1 ml Simplastin add 0.4 ml normal saline to make a 1:5 dilution.
4. Make 1:50 and 1:500 dilutions by serial dilution of this 1:5 dilution.
5. Place 0.1 ml of the 1:50 dilution in a glass test tube and add 0.1 ml patient's plasma. Incubate for 5 minutes at 37°C.
6. Blow in 0.1 ml calcium chloride solution and start a timer simultaneously.
7. Determine the clotting time and repeat with a second tube.
8. Repeat steps 4 through 6, using patient's plasma and the 1:500 dilution of Simplastin.
9. Perform the same procedure on a normal control plasma, using the 1:50 and 1:500 dilutions of Simplastin.
10. Calculate the ratio of the clotting time of the patient's plasma and the normal control plasma:

$$\frac{\text{patient PT}}{\text{control PT}}$$

Normal Values: Less than 1.1 is normal ratio; 1.1 to 1.3 is borderline; greater than 1.3 is diagnostic of the lupus anticoagulant (Table 12-2).

Reference

Schleider MA, et al: A clinical study of the lupus anticoagulant. Blood 48:499, 1976.

HEPARIN ASSAY
(Synthetic Fluorogenic-Substrate)

In this assay, heparin is measured indirectly by adding diluted pooled normal plasma to a heparinized plasma sample and measuring residual thrombin activity on a synthetic fluorogenic-substrate after the addition of a known amount of thrombin. The normal plasma makes available normal amounts of antithrombin III, which eliminates this variable that may influence the anticoagulant effect of heparin as measured by clotting tests. This is, therefore, a measure of the level of circulating heparin but not necessarily its anticoagulant effect in the patient's plasma.

Equipment

1. Protopath fluorometer (Dade, Miami, FL).
2. Plastic test tubes, 12 × 75 mm.
3. Pipettes that can measure 5.0 ml, 2.0 ml, 1.0 ml, 0.5 ml, 0.2 ml, 0.05 ml and 5 μl.
4. 37°C heating block or water bath.
5. Vortex mixer.
6. Stopwatch.

Reagents

1. Protopath Heparin Synthetic Substrate Assay Kit (Dade).
   a. Lyophilized diluted citrated plasma reagent (1:40 dilution). Store at 2

to 8°C. Reconstitute with 5.0 ml distilled water, restopper vial, and swirl gently until dissolved. Store at 2 to 8°C when not in use. Discard after 7 days.

b.   Lyophilized thrombin reagent (human). Store at 2 to 8°C. Reconstitute with 1.0 ml distilled water, restopper vial, and swirl gently until dissolved. Maintain at 2 to 8°C or in ice bath (when in use). Discard after 72 hours. (Do not use glass pipettes for measuring thrombin reagent.)

c.   Thrombin substrate. A lyophilized preparation of 0.3 μmoles D-phenylalanine-proline-arginine-AIE in buffer-containing stabilizers, in disposable cuvettes packaged in a foil pouch. Substrate is identified by a red dot on the cuvette. Store at 2 to 8°C. Reconstitute with 2.0 ml distilled water to give a concentration of 0.15 μmoles per ml substrate. After reconstitution, substrate is stable for 4 hours at room temperature or 8 hours stored at 2 to 8°C. Protect from light.

d.   Heparin control. A lyophilized, citrated human plasma pool with sodium heparin added. Assayed value is on first page of package insert. Store at 2 to 8°C. Reconstitute with 0.5 ml distilled water, restopper vial, and swirl gently until dissolved. Store at 2 to 8°C when not in use. Discard after 8 hours.

2.   Heparin (1,000 USP units per ml). Same source as the heparin used for patient therapy.

3.   Pooled normal plasma. Freshly collected, citrated normal plasma from 4 to 10 donors for preparation of the heparin standard curve. (Collect and prepare as for patient's samples).

4.   Sodium citrate solution (3.8%).

5.   Normal saline (0.85%).

Procedure

Collection of Specimens

1.   Obtain blood from patient and add 4.5 ml to 0.5 ml sodium citrate solution.

2.   Centrifuge sample for 10 minutes at 3000 rpm and remove plasma.

3.   Store plasma in a plastic tube at 2 to 8°C until assayed. Assay within 8 hours.

Note: Time of collection is important since the in vivo half-life of heparin is approximately 1.5 hours. Platelet factor 4, a heparin-neutralizing platelet factor, can be released from platelets, so blood should be collected with a minimum of trauma, preferably using a plastic syringe or an evacuated tube, if extreme caution is taken. Care should be taken to assure adequate centrifugation of both the patient's blood and that used for the normal plasma pool.

Preparation of Dilutions for Heparin Standard Curve

1.   Turn on the Protopath Fluorometer and leave sample-compartment cover closed. Allow approximately 45 minutes for the instrument to reach 37°C before use.

2. Place several 12 × 75 mm plastic test tubes in the heating block or water bath to prewarm to 37°C.
3. Prepare a stock solution of heparin to a final concentration of 80 USP per ml in normal saline. (Add 1.0 ml of 1000 USP units/ml to 11.5 ml of saline.)
4. Prepare heparin standards by diluting the stock heparin solution (80 units/ml) in the plasma pool as follows:
   a. 0.1 ml stock + 0.9 ml plasma = 8 units/ml standard (not assayed).
   b. 0.1 ml 8 units/ml standard + 0.9 ml plasma = 0.8 units/ml standard.
   c. 0.5 ml 0.8 unit/ml standard + 0.5 ml plasma = 0.4 unit/ml standard.
   d. 0.5 ml 0.4 unit/ml standard + 0.5 ml plasma = 0.2 units/ml standard.
   e. 0.5 ml 0.2 unit/ml standard + 0.5 ml plasma = 0.1 unit/ml standard.
   f. 0.5 ml plasma = zero standard (heparin assay blank).

Discard 8 units/ml standard and store remaining heparinized normal plasma standards (including the zero standard) at 2 to 8°C until ready to use. Discard after 1 day.

Calibration of Heparin Assay Blank (Zero Standard)

1. With distilled water, reconstitute the required number of vials of citrated plasma (24 tests per vial) and thrombin reagent (19 tests per vial). Maintain thrombin at 2 to 8°C (in ice bath when in use). If more than one vial is reconstituted, pool before use.
2. Reconstitute one vial of heparin control.
3. Reconstitute one thrombin-substrate cuvette for each blank (zero standard), 4 heparin standards, heparin control, and patient's sample to be tested. Do not invert cuvettes after reconstitution.
4. Warm cuvette in the heating block of the protopath fluorometer for at least 10 minutes before using, but not for more than 1 hour. Do not place in light path until test mixture is added. Protect reconstituted substrate from direct light.
5. Check and calibrate the instrument according to instructions for its operation.
6. To test the zero standard:
   a. Pipette 0.2 ml citrated plasma reagent into a prewarmed test tube. Allow 1 to 2 minutes for reagent to reach 37°C.
   b. Pipette 5 μl pooled normal plasma containing no heparin (zero standard) into the test tube containing citrated plasma reagent.
   c. Add 0.05 ml thrombin reagent to the tube and simultaneously start the stopwatch. Mix by rinsing pipette tip several times in the reagent.
   d. After exactly 60 seconds, pour the contents of a prewarmed cuvette into the test tube. Immediately pour the reaction mixture back into the cuvette. Note: If lung rather than mucosal heparin is being used, increase the incubation time to 120 seconds.
   e. Place the cuvette in the sample well of the fluorometer and close the sample-compartment cover.
   f. Press the READ on the touch panel. The digital display will flash on and off. The reading is taken when the flashing stops.

g. For the heparin assay blank, the value displayed should be 100 ± 5. If the value is not 100 ± 5, repeat the blank. If the repeat value is still not 100 ± 5, adjust the calibrator control for test selector A, according to instructions for the fluorometer.

Testing for Heparin

1. Test heparin standards (0.8 U/ml, 0.4 U/ml, 0.2 U/ml, 0.1 U/ml) in the same way as the zero standard and record the digital readouts taken when the flashing stops.
2. Then test the heparin control supplied with the kit, and the patient's samples.

Determination of Results

1. Plot the value of percent thrombin remaining for each heparin standard on the ordinate, and the corresponding heparin concentration on the abscissa of linear graph paper.
2. Heparin concentration values for the heparin control and the patient's samples are read directly from the standard curve.
3. Heparin concentration for the heparin control should correspond to the recorded value in the package insert.
4. If patient's samples contain more than 0.8 U/ml heparin, dilute appropriately in pooled, freshly collected, citrated normal plasma and retest. Multiply the value obtained by the dilution factor.

Normal Ranges: Values obtained for normal plasma from patients not receiving heparin therapy should be the same as the blank's value. The heparin concentrations and the range for heparin standards determined by using USP Reference Standard Heparin and the synthetic fluorogenic-substrate method described are given below:

USP unit/ml	Mean ± 2SD
0.1	82 ± 6
0.2	65 ± 6
0.4	42 ± 10
0.8	20 ± 10

References

Protopath Proteolytic Enzyme Detection System. Heparin Synthetic Substrate Assay, package insert. Miami, Dade, 1979.
Triplett DA, and Harms C: The use of the fluorogenic synthetic substrate assay for the clinical determination of heparin. Thromb Haemost 42:308, 1979.

PROTAMINE SULFATE TITRATION FOR HEPARIN ACTIVITY

Reagents

1. Sodium citrate (3.8%), sodium oxalate (0.1 *M*), or acid-citrate solution.
2. Barbital-buffered saline.
3. Protamine sulfate (1% solution).
4. Thrombin solution. A stock solution may be made by adding 10 ml 50% glycerol in barbital-buffered saline to a vial containing 1000 units bovine

topical thrombin and stored in the freezer. This solution can be further diluted with normal control plasma to give a thrombin time of 10 to 15 seconds (approximately 5 U/ml).

5.   Normal control plasma (freshly prepared, commercial standard normal plasma).

Procedure

1.   Draw 4.5 ml patient's blood and add it to 0.5 ml anticoagulant solution. Vacutainers may be used.
2.   Centrifuge for 10 minutes at 3000 rpm and remove the plasma.
3.   Determine the thrombin time of 0.1 ml control plasma plus 0.1 ml barbital-buffered saline by adding 0.1 ml thrombin solution to this mixture.
4.   Dilute protamine sulfate as follows in numbered tubes:

      (1)   1.0 ml 1% protamine + 99 ml barbital-buffered saline
             = 100 μg/ml
      (2)   0.5 ml of (1) + 4.5 ml barbital-buffered saline = 10 μg/ml
      (3)   2.0 ml of (2) + 2.0 ml barbital-buffered saline = 5 μg/ml
      (4)   2.0 ml of (3) + 2.0 ml barbital-buffered saline = 2.5 μg/ml
      (5)   2.0 ml of (4) + 2.0 ml barbital-buffered saline = 1.25 μg/ml

5.   Pipette 0.1 ml patient's plasma into each of 5 numbered tubes and add 0.1 ml protamine solution from each of the 5 dilutions to the appropriate tube.
6.   Add 0.1 ml thrombin solution to each and determine the clotting time.
7.   Determine the lowest concentration of protamine that gives a thrombin time equal to that of the normal control plasma as determined in step 3.

Interpretation

The amount of protamine sulfate required to neutralize heparin activity can be calculated as follows: Since the test determines the neutralizing dose of protamine per ml plasma, the μg/ml protamine required should be multiplied by the estimated plasma volume of the patient to determine the total dose needed.

APPENDIX

I. EQUIPMENT

Needles

Disposable needles should be used. If quantities of 10 to 15 ml of blood are to be drawn, the No. 20 and No. 21 needles are adequate; but for larger quantities, the No. 19 is probably more satisfactory. Siliconized needles (Scientific Products—S9540) are available for use with plastic syringes and are preferred for drawing blood for platelet studies.

Syringes

In most instances, syringes should be of the disposable plastic type and should be used only once. The two-syringe technique should be utilized whenever a group of tests is to be done because of the danger of contaminating blood in the first syringe with tissue thromboplastin. Blood from the first syringe may be used for clot retraction, prothrombin time, thrombin time, and clot lysis tests. Blood from the second syringe should be reserved for the partial thromboplastin times, prothrombin consumption test, thromboplastin generation tests, and assays for factors VIII, IX, and the contact factors.

Vacutainers

Regular Vacutainers containing sodium oxalate (0.1 M) or sodium citrate (3.8%) may be used for the collection of blood, providing the tube to be used for clotting studies is the second tube to be drawn. VACUTAINER Brand Coag tubes are available from Becton Dickinson Co. These have a "non-wettable" tube lining, which minimizes glass activation, and are available with 3.2% or 3.8% buffered sodium citrate. We always use siliconized Vacutainers with 3.8% sodium citrate to collect blood for platelet function studies and sometimes for other testing. Care must be used with Vacutainers to be sure that the proper quantity of blood is drawn into the tube. Sometimes the vacuum is faulty originally, or it may become decreased on storage of the tubes. It is well to note in advance the exact point on the tube that should be reached when 4.5 ml blood are mixed with the 0.5 ml anticoagulant. Maintaining a constant ratio of anticoagulant to blood is important in the accuracy and reproducibility of coagulation tests. When foaming occurs during the use of Vacutainers, factors I, V, and VIII may be denatured. Vacutainers containing EDTA may be used to draw blood for platelet counts but not for any other coagulation tests, except the quantitative fibrinogen assay and some immunologic procedures.

Test Tubes

Plastic Tubes. It is advisable to collect and store blood for most tests in plastic tubes. The 13 × 100 mm size is convenient for the collection of 4.5 ml blood in 0.5 ml anticoagulant. After separation, the plasma also is preferably stored in plastic tubes (12 × 75 mm) in the refrigerator or ice bath until time for coagulation testing. Since it is obvious that surface activation takes place in the absence of calcium, it is possible for many changes to occur in the blood or plasma standing in glass tubes. Such changes are minimized by the use of plastic syringes and tubes or siliconized Vacutainers for initial handling of the blood and plasma. Platelet-rich plasma for platelet function tests should be stored in plastic tubes at room temperature.

Glass Tubes. Plain glass tubes may be used for all the remaining coagulation tests. One size should be selected and used for clotting tests. Tubes 12 × 75 mm are a convenient size. Larger tubes may be required for incubation mixtures in two-stage tests. Disposable glass tubes are preferable. If tubes are to be reused, they should be used exclusively for coagulation tests and not circulated through departments of the laboratory. They should be cleaned carefully with a good laboratory detergent, rinsed about 20 times, the final rinsings being with distilled water, and then dried in an oven. They should be inspected regularly and discarded if scratched, because the scratched tube may result in unequal surface activation besides interfering with accurate detection of the end point of clotting. Acid cleaning of test tubes that are to be used in coagulation studies is unnecessary, and repeated exposure to chromic-acid cleaning solution may result in tubes that have a non-wettable surface similar to that of silicone. With the increasing use of activated procedures such as the APTT, the character and condition of the glassware has become less and less important.

Pipettes

Pipetting by mouth should be avoided whenever possible because of the danger of accidental infection or damage to the pipetter. Automatic pipetting devices which utilize disposable plastic tips are highly satisfactory. Many systems are available with varied precalibrated volume selectors which include commonly used volumes from 1 μl to 1.0 ml. Disposable tips eliminate the need for cleaning pipettes and prevent cross-contamination between samples. The potential for human error is also reduced. Most automatic coagulation instruments include automatic pipettes. For pipetting the larger volumes used in the preparation of reagents, standard graduated glass pipettes should be used.

Automatic Instruments

Many automatic clot timer instruments are available. Each laboratory should make selections that fit its specific needs and should become thoroughly acquainted with the use of each instrument that is chosen. We use the following instruments, which give us a good range of adaptability for testing single and multiple samples.

1. The *Fibrometer* (BBL Microbiology System) is a semiautomated instrument that is satisfactory for many clotting end-point tests. The instrument contains a thermal heating block which holds disposable plastic containers for testing. An automatic pipette dispenses plasma and reagents and starts the time cycle automatically. Clot formation is recorded by an electromechanical fibrin switch. The Fibrometer is not entirely satisfactory for the partial thromboplastin time and for the one-stage assays based on this test because of carry-over of coagulation substances on the probe when it is not cleaned carefully after each test.

2. The *Coagulation Profiler* (Bio/Data Corp.) provides a semiautomated system which is either single or dual channelled. It operates on a photo-optical principle in which the rate of change of optical density is measured electronically. In operation, test plasma is placed in a test tube and inserted into the sample well of the instrument. The final reagent added to the test plasma initiates the timer. Light received through the test sample by a photo detector is converted into electronic signals, amplified and differentiated for end-point detection (digital readout). The Bio/Data Profiler system also provides a graphic illustration (thrombokinetogram) of the entire coagulation process by automatically recording both the kinetics of fibrin formation and the degree of change in optical density. The latter information relates particularly to the concentration of fibrinogen, since higher levels of fibrinogen cause greater changes in optical density. This instrument can be used for all clotting end-point tests.

3. The *Coag-A-Mate* (General Diagnostics) single- and dual-channel instruments also operate on a photo-optical clot-detection system for the fully automatic determination of prothrombin times and other related coagulation tests. A plastic filter surrounds the light source and provides a uniform light beam through the sample cuvette. A second filter is located in front of the electro-optical sensor. This sensor instantly converts the transmitted light into an electrical signal that is amplified, compared, and conditioned to control the time-display circuit. In operation, samples are placed in a disposable circular test tray, which is then placed on the incubation test plate of the instrument. When the test cycle is started, a pump automatically delivers the reagent that initiates the clotting reaction and, simultaneously, the electronic clock is activated. A test-mode selector and cycle-time control allow adjustments to accommodate those tests that require preincubation, such as the APTT. Clot formation is detected by a rate of change in absorbance that exceeds a predetermined level for a defined period of time.

Extended or prolonged clotting times pose problems for all automated instruments, but particularly for instruments that employ photo-optical systems. The rate of clotting may be slow and the formed clot of such poor quality that the instrument does not detect the clot and fails to deactivate or stop the timer. Laboratories should routinely establish a point at which all prolonged values are rechecked by a manual method.

II. REAGENTS

Acetic Acid (1%)

Dilute 1.0 ml concentrated acetic acid to 100 ml distilled water. This is used to acidify the plasma in precipitating out the euglobulin fraction in the euglobulin clot lysis test.

Adenosine Diphosphate (ADP)

The disodium salt of adenosine-5'-diphosphate is available from Sigma Chemical Co. Dissolve 11.8 mg in 10 ml barbital buffer to make stock solution and dilute further to make "strong" or "weak" solutions for platelet aggregation tests.

Adrenalin Chloride

Adrenalin chloride is available from Parke-Davis in 30 ml vials (1 mg/ml) and is diluted 0.1 ml to 1.82 ml with normal saline to test for platelet aggregation. It is also used in the direct method for measuring PF_3 in a concentration of 1 mg/ml.

Adsorbants and Adsorbed Plasma Reagents

Several insoluble salts and bases remove factor II and other clotting factors by adsorption. The two most commonly used are barium sulfate ($BaSO_4$) and aluminum hydroxide ($AL (OH)_2$), which act on plasma in the following way:

Adsorbed (in Eluate)	Not Adsorbed (in Plasma)
Factor II	Factor I
Factor VII	Factor V
Factor IX	Factor XI
Factor X	Factor XII

They can be used interchangeably, except that barium sulfate cannot be used with citrated plasma. Each laboratory should decide on one adsorbant and use it for all tests that require adsorbed plasma or serum. This decision will certainly be influenced by the choice of the routine anticoagulant. If citrate is to be used routinely, then the adsorbant should be aluminum hydroxide.

1. To adsorb oxalated plasma chemically-pure, powdered barium sulfate is mixed with the plasma in a proportion of 100 mg/ml. This mixture is allowed to stand at room temperature for 10 minutes, with intermittent agitation. It is then centrifuged for 10 minutes, and the upper three fourths of the plasma is decanted and stored in the refrigerator until used.
2. Aluminum hydroxide gel may be purchased as Alhydrox (Cutter) or unflavored Amphogel (Wyeth). It should be used in the proportion of 0.1 ml/ml citrated or oxalated plasma. The mixture is stirred at 37°C for 3 minutes and then centrifuged for 5 minutes. The upper three fourths of the plasma is decanted and stored in the refrigerator until used.

The prothrombin time for such adsorbed plasmas should be over 5 minutes. Adsorbed plasma contains factors I, V, VIII, XI, and XII. It is used in the thromboplastin generation test, in the differential activated partial thromboplastin time, and in the differential prothrombin time. If the adsorbant is eluted, the eluate will contain factors II, VII, IX, and X. Adsorbed plasma reagent is commercially available from Dade, George King, and General Diagnostics.

Arachidonic Acid

This reagent is available from Bio/Data in 0.5 ml vials for use in platelet aggregation testing.

Anticoagulants

It is probably advisable for each laboratory to adopt a single anticoagulant to be used for all routine coagulation procedures. Both sodium oxalate and sodium citrate are satisfactory, but sodium citrate is used by most investigators and is preferable in some procedures. Plasma clotting times are usually somewhat shorter when citrate is used. Factors V and VIII are better preserved with citrate, and the plasma may be stored somewhat longer before being tested; however, factors II, VII, and X are enhanced with storage in citrate. When barium sulfate is to be used as an adsorbant, the plasma must be oxalated rather than citrated. Either oxalated or citrated plasma may be used with aluminum hydroxide as an adsorbant. Heparin has no place as an anticoagulant in coagulation tests, but it is used in the collection of blood to be tested for platelet retention in glass bead columns.

Preparation of Sodium Oxalate Solutions

To prepare 0.1 M sodium oxalate solution, 1.34 g/100 ml distilled water is used. Sodium oxalate solution removes calcium from the blood because of differences in the solubility products of sodium oxalate and calcium oxalate. The solution should be filtered before use and kept in the refrigerator in order to retard growth of mold. If barium sulfate is used for adsorption of plasma, sodium oxalate should be used as the anticoagulant. The proportion of blood to oxalate is 9 ml to 1 ml. When sodium oxalate is used as the anticoagulant, the oxalate forms a cloudy suspension when calcium is added during clotting tests, giving a sharp, opaque end point.

Preparation of Sodium Citrate Solutions

Various concentrations of sodium citrate solution have been suggested, ranging from 2.95% (0.1 M) to 3.8% (0.129 M), but each laboratory should adopt a single concentration. The 3.8% solution, which is prepared by adding 3.8 g sodium citrate to 100 ml distilled water, has been the most frequently recommended, and this is what we use. The International Committee for Standardization in Hematology has recently adopted 3.2% buffered sodium-citrate as the standard for coagulation studies. One volume of citrate to 9 volumes of blood is the correct proportion. Citrate solutions should be filtered and stored in the refrigerator to retard the growth of mold. The 3.8% solution may be used as a diluent for platelet counts if it is filtered before each use.

Acid-citrate solutions can also be used. Such reagents contain sodium citrate and citric acid to give a lower pH. The activated partial thromboplastin time is definitely shorter when such anticoagulants are used. The reason for selecting a buffered-citrate anticoagulant is that the pH of the plasma holds constant for a longer period of time.

The use of buffered APTT reagents has decreased the importance of this anticoagulant.

Considerable evidence exists that the primary anticoagulant action of citrate is not a depression of ionized calcium but a direct action on the prothrombin molecule, although at higher concentrations, depression of calcium ions also occurs. This may explain the wide variation in recommended concentrations and the suggestion by some workers that citrated plasma should be allowed to stand at least 15 minutes and perhaps longer before testing it. Because citrate forms a soluble complex with calcium when sodium citrate is used as the anticoagulant, the end point of plasma clotting tests is not as sharp as with oxalate.

Preparation of Disodium Ethylenediaminetetraacetate (EDTA)

The dry reagent is used in proportion of 1 mg/ml blood. This anticoagulant acts solely by removing or depressing ionized calcium and may be used in the collection of blood for platelet counts. It should not be employed for any coagulation tests, except the quantitative fibrinogen assay when it is preferred because of the elimination of the dilution factor. It retards the clotting time of the thrombin-fibrinogen system, and the tensile strength of the clot formed from EDTA plasma is greatly reduced. It prevents clumping of platelets, and if smears are made from blood mixed with EDTA, useful information about the number and size of platelet clumps cannot be obtained.

Preparation of Ammonium Oxalate Solution

The concentration of ammonium oxalate solution to be used for platelet-count diluent is 1%. It is used for platelet counts because it is both an anticoagulant and a hemolytic agent. The solution is likely to show bacterial growth and should be stored in the refrigerator and filtered before each use. Dilution may be made in an erythrocyte-counting pipette, where the dilution factor is 1:200. It is more convenient, however, to use the Unopette (Becton Dickinson Co.), a disposable blood-dilution pipette with a carefully measured amount of 1% ammonium oxalate in a plastic container. This pipette is satisfactory for platelet and leukocyte counts. The dilution factor is 1:100 instead of the 1:200 of the erythrocyte-counting pipette.

Buffers and Buffered Saline

There has been little uniformity in the choice of buffers for coagulation studies, and many tests appear to work very well unbuffered. It is probably desirable, however, to buffer coagulation reactions to a pH within the physiologic range of approximately 7.34 to 7.43. This is particularly important when procedures call for significant dilutions of reagents or plasma. Unbuffered normal saline solutions that are stored in the laboratory, even when tightly capped, tend to show marked variation in pH and usually have pH values well below 7.0. For this reason, we use buffered saline as a diluent for all clotting tests and have found either barbital-buffered saline or tris-buffered saline satisfactory.

When it is necessary to dilute whole blood, it is important to have an isotonic solution that will not disrupt the red cells, because coagulant material may be released. The phosphate buffer recommended for the diluted whole-blood fibrinolysis test has an ionic strength of 0.15, which is essentially isotonic. It cannot, however, be used in tests that require the addition of calcium, because phosphate is incompatible with calcium salts.

Michaelis acetate-barbital-buffered saline has a pH of 7.42 and an ionic strength of approximately 0.15, and imidizole-buffered saline may be prepared to have a pH of 7.25 and ionic strength of 0.14. Even though these are more nearly isotonic, they have no advantages over barbital-buffered saline or tris-buffered saline for plasma clotting tests. All buffer solutions should be refrigerated.

1. *Barbital-buffered saline* is recommended for most of the tests described in this book. It has a pH of 7.35 and an ionic strength of approximately 0.10. It is commercially available or can be prepared by adding 11.75 g sodium diethylbarbiturate and 14.67 g sodium chloride to 1570 ml distilled water and then adding 430 ml 0.1 N hydrochloric acid. This should give a final pH of 7.35. It is stable indefinitely at refrigerator temperatures.

2. *Tris buffer or tris-buffered saline* is inexpensive and can also be used for all types of plasma coagulation tests. It is known not to inhibit enzyme reactions. Its buffering power is somewhat low at pH 7.4, but it is adequate for dilute plasma tests. Its pH is somewhat dependent on temperature, being lower at 37°C than at room temperature. The ionic strength of tris-buffered saline is approximately 0.09. A stock solution of tris base can be made by dissolving 24.3 g tris base $NH_2C(CH_2OH)$ in 1000 ml distilled water. Combine 250 ml of this and 42 ml 1 N hydrochloric acid and dilute to 990 ml with distilled water. Add 2.2 g sodium chloride and adjust the pH to 7.4 at room temperature. The final volume is made up to 1000 ml with distilled water. Both this buffer and tris-buffered saline are commerically available from Sigma Chemical Co.

3. *Phosphate buffer* is used for the diluted whole-blood clot fibrinolysis test. It is prepared by dissolving 9.47 g disodium phosphate in 1000 ml distilled water. To this solution is added 250 ml monopotassium phosphate solution prepared by dissolving 3.02 g KH_2PO_4 in 250 ml distilled water. The solution should be sterilized before refrigeration.

4. *Borate buffer* is used in the ethanol gelation test. It has a pH of 8.0 and is 0.15 *M*. A stock solution is made up of boric acid 0.15 *M* and sodium borate 0.15 *M* mixed to achieve a pH of 8. This is then mixed with ethanol to make the borate buffer/ethanol reagent.

5. *Buffered EDTA solution* is used for the platelet-count-ratio method for the quantitation of platelet aggregates. It is made by adding 3 ml of 0.77 *M* EDTA and 5 ml concentrated phosphate-buffered saline (2 g KCl, 2 g KH_2PO_4, 80 g NaCl, and 17.3 g $Na_2HPO_4 \cdot 7H_2O$ in 1000 ml distilled water) to 12 ml of distilled water. The pH is 7.26 and the osmolality, 700 mOsm/L.

Reference

Gomori G: Buffers in the range of pH 6.5 to 9.6. Proc Soc Exp Biol 62:33, 1946.

Calcium Chloride Solution

Calcium solutions are required generally as a source of calcium ions in the clotting process, but some of the early contact-activation reactions take place in the absence of these ions. The thrombin-fibrinogen reaction can also occur in the absence of calcium. A 0.02 M calcium chloride solution is thought to be ideal for the shortest coagulation time of decalcified blood when the test is carried out in plain glassware. There seems to be little reason for the variation in the concentrations that are required for the different tests, except that the reported normal results have been obtained by the use of the specified concentration. We would suggest that each laboratory adopt one concentration and use it for all tests. If the concentration is altered in a given procedure, normal values should be established for the concentration used, and reported with the test results by the individual laboratory. The most frequently recommended concentrations are the following:

1. 0.02 M, prepared by dissolving 0.222 g anhydrous calcium chloride in 100 ml distilled water.
2. 0.025 M, prepared by dissolving 0.277 g anhydrous calcium in 100 ml distilled water.
3. 0.5 M, prepared by dissolving 5.55 g anhydrous calcium chloride in 100 ml distilled water (for use in the thrombin generation time test).

We have elected to use 0.025 M for all standard clotting tests, and we store the solution in the refrigerator to retard growth of mold. The 0.025 M solution was selected to allow for increased concentrations of anticoagulant which occur when patients have high hematocrit values.

Collagen Suspension

Collagen is available from Sigma Chemical Co. A suspension is prepared with modified Tyrode's solution, as described in the procedure for platelet aggregation testing (page 93).

Contact Activators

These substances may be incubated with plasma to bring about maximum surface activation of the "contact system" and thus reduce variations in the results of clotting tests that are due to differences in exposure of plasma to glass surfaces.

1. *Kaolin* (china clay, Braun Chemical Co.) is a white powder usually dissolved in normal saline in the proportion of 0.5 to 2.0 g/100 ml saline. It may be incubated with plasma in the performance of the activated partial thromboplastin time test. Kaolin is also used in the platelet-factor-3-availability test.
2. *Celite* (Johns Manville Co.) is a diatomaceous silica, usually suspended in normal saline solution or buffered saline in the proportion of 3 to 5 g/100 ml. It may also be incubated with plasma in the activated partial thromboplastin time test. Micronized silica is used in some APTT reagents (General Diagnostics).
3. *Ellagic acid* is a chemical surface-activator. It is present in APTT reagents from Dade and Ortho Diagnostics.

References

Margolis J: The Kaolin clotting time. J Clin Pathol 11:406, 1958.
Proctor RP, and Rapaport SI: The partial thromboplastin time with kaolin. Am J Clin Pathol 36:212, 1961.

Control Plasma

Standardized, lyophilized control plasmas considered to be 100% normal for use in the prothrombin time (PT) and activated partial thromboplastin time tests (APTT), are available from most manufacturers who make coagulation reagents. Some are prepared from pools of oxalated plasma and some from citrated plasma. The prothrombin time test shows little difference in the normal values obtained with control plasmas from different manufacturers. This is not true, however, for the partial thromboplastin time tests. Some manufacturers have elected to prepare a control plasma that regularly gives a partial thromboplastin time at the lower end of the normal range, whereas others market control plasmas with values closer to the upper limit of normal. It is important to have this information about the particular product selected. The control plasma selected should be provided by the manufacturer of the selected PT and APTT reagents. Most control plasmas have been assayed for a variety of coagulation factors.

Abnormal coagulation control plasmas, low in factors II, VII, IX, and X, are available from several manufacturers and are designed to give values in the prothrombin time test that are two to three times normal. This allows the laboratory to determine whether the reagents being used are reacting as expected with abnormal plasma.

Normal plasma pools can be collected, frozen, and stored in aliquots at $-20°C$ for use as control plasma in many coagulation tests. A frozen-plasma pool that has been assayed for most clotting factors is also available from some manufacturers (George King-Bio-Medical).

Fibrinogen reference plasma is a dried human plasma that has been treated and standardized to give reproducible fibrinogen values. Such reference plasmas are used to make a standard curve for the determination of fibrinogen by the Clauss method and in preparing a positive fibrinogen control for the staphylococcal clumping test.

Epsilon Aminocaproic Acid (EACA, Amicar)

EACA acts both in vitro and in vivo as an inhibitor of fibrinolysis. It is available from Lederle in 20 ml vials, containing 250 mg/ml. A 1.0 M solution is added to blood that is to be tested for fibrinogen-fibrin degradation products (FDP) in the staphylococcal clumping test; and is used in the serial-dilution protamine saline test. A solution containing 18 mg/2 drops (Sigma Chemical Co.) can also be used for the collection of serum for FDP tests.

Factor-Deficient Substrate Plasmas

Specific-factor-deficient substrates are used in assay procedures for the various factors. Most are available lyophilized from Dade, General Diagnostics, and Helena Laboratories and frozen from George King-Bio-Medical.

1. *Factor II-Deficient Substrate Plasma.* A satisfactory prothrombin-deficient substrate plasma may be made by combining equal parts of adsorbed plasma and oxalated serum.

2. *Factor V-Deficient Substrate Plasma.* When plasma is stored for 2 weeks at 5°C or 24 hours at 37°C, it becomes deficient in factor V. The prothrombin time of such a plasma should be over 25 seconds.

3. *Factor VII-Deficient Substrate Plasma.* This is a plasma from a patient known to be almost completely deficient in factor VII.

4. *Factor X-Deficient Substrate Plasma.* This is a plasma from a patient known to be almost completely deficient in factor X.

5. *Factor VII-and-X-Deficient Substrate Plasma.* This reagent may be prepared by using a Seitz filter and fresh 30% asbestos filter pads to filter 100 ml bovine plasma by suction. The pressure should be low to avoid foaming. The first 20 ml should be discarded; the remaining 80 ml will be found to contain fibrinogen, factor V, and about 60% of factor II, but to lack factors VII and X. This reagent may be stored in aliquots in the freezer for a year. Dried reagent is available from Sigma Chemical Co.

6. *Factor VIII-Deficient Substrate Plasma.* This is plasma from a patient known to be almost completely deficient in factor VIII. When such patients are regularly available, it may be possible to obtain blood from them at intervals. If such blood is drawn carefully, and the plasma is separated promptly and frozen in aliquots, it is satisfactory for use for varying periods of time, probably up to 3 months.

7. *Factor IX-Deficient Substrate Plasma.* Plasma from a known factor IX-deficient patient may be collected and stored in the same way suggested for plasma from a factor VIII-deficient patient.

8. *Factor XI- and Factor XII-Deficient Plasma or Serum.* Factor XI may be removed by incubating 1 ml plasma or serum with 15 mg celite. If the quantity of celite is increased to 30 mg/ml, both factors XI and XII are removed by adsorption on the celite. Factor XI may be destroyed in serum by heating to 56°C for 30 minutes. Factor XII is more heat-stable, and it remains active unless the serum is further heated to 60°C for 30 minutes. Since fibrinogen is precipitated at 56°C, it is not practical to heat plasma to separate these factors.

9. *Prekallikrein (Fletcher),-high molecular weight kininogen (Fitzgerald)- and Passavoy-deficient plasmas* are available frozen from George King-Bio-Medical.

10. *von Willebrand-deficient plasma* is available frozen from George King-Bio-Medical.

Fibrinogen

Dried bovine-fibrinogen is available from Sigma Chemical Co. (5, 10, 25, 50 g) and General Diagnostics (300 mg/vial). The dried fibrinogen must be reconstituted with distilled water or buffered saline to give a specific concentration. In the dry form it is stable indefinitely at refrigerator temperature, but the solution is stable for only 12 hours at 5°C and 24 hours at room temperature. This reagent may be used in the prothrombin consumption test and in tests for fibrinolysis when the patient's fibrinogen level is decreased. It is also used in the clotting test for antithrombin III.

Formaldehyde

A 2% concentration of formaldehyde is used to treat platelets for the measurement of factor VIIIR : WF. A 4% concentration is used to make the buffered EDTA-formalin solution for the quantitation of platelet aggregates.

Heparin

Heparin is available from several manufacturers in vials of 1000 USP units/ml. It is added to plasma in varying amounts to prepare a heparin control curve for use in monitoring heparin therapy. The heparin chosen should be that supplied by the same manufacturer that supplies the material used to treat patients served by the laboratory. Heparin is also used as an anticoagulant in the collection of blood for testing platelet retention in glass bead columns at a concentration of 4 U/ml whole blood.

Phenol Reagent (Folin-Ciocalteu)

This reagent is used only in the fibrinogen assay procedure (pages 163 and 165).

Partial Thromboplastins and Activated Partial Thromboplastins

Partial thromboplastins are lipid reagents that are used as substitutes for platelets in clotting tests and include the following:
1. Chloroform extract of rabbit brain made by the method of Bell and Alton. Commercial products that contain only partial thromboplastin reagent made in this manner include Platelin (General Diagnostics) and Thrombofax (Ortho).
2. Inosithin (Associated Concentrates, Inc.). This commercial soybean-phospholipid is usually prepared by making a 5% stock solution of 1.25 g in 25 ml buffered saline. This may be further diluted as needed.

Activated partial thromboplastins are mixtures of contact activators (kaolin, micronized silica, or ellagic acid) and lipid partial thromboplastins and are used to perform the activated partial thromboplastin time and other coagulation tests. The purpose of using the combination is to substitute for, and thus minimize, the two major variables of contact activation and platelet numbers in testing the plasma coagulation system. Several of these reagents are commercially available. It is important to realize that considerable variation exists in these reagents and that the results using different reagents are not strictly comparable. Therefore, one product should be selected and used consistently. If results show unusual variation with a given reagent, it is wise to check samples with a different reagent system. We have seen extreme variations, using different reagents with a single sample, especially when the reagents contain different types of activators.

Platelet-Aggregation Reagents

These are available in kits from Dade, Bio/Data and Pacific Hemostasis Laboratories.

Platelet-rich Plasma

This may be obtained when blood is drawn in anticoagulant and centrifuged for 10 minutes at 1000 rpm. Plasma should be removed immediately. A yield of 60% platelets calculated from the whole-blood platelet count is adequate.

Platelet-poor Plasma

This is obtained when blood is drawn in anticoagulant and centrifuged for 10 minutes at 3000 rpm or for 5 minutes at 15,000 rpm. Plasma should be removed immediately.

Polybrene

Polybrene neutralizes the anticoagulant action of heparin. It is available from Aldrich in 10-gram vials and is used in the serum AT III-activity test to neutralize heparin; the stock solution is 10 mg/ml normal saline and the working solution is .005 mg/ml normal saline.

Protamine Sulfate (1% Solution)

Protamine sulfate neutralizes the anticoagulant action of heparin and also produces a paracoagulation reaction when soluble fibrin monomer complexes are present in plasma. It is available from Lilly in ampoules which contain a 1% solution (50 mg/5 ml). This should be stored in the refrigerator. It is used in the serial-dilution protamine sulfate test and in the protamine sulfate titration for heparin activity.

Ristocetin

Ristocetin is an antibiotic that is useful in testing platelet aggregation, especially in the diagnosis of von Willebrand's disease. It is also used in the factor VIIIR:WF assay. It is available from Bio/Data and Helena Laboratories.

Russell's Viper Venom (Stypven)

This is a thromboplastin substance that also has factor VII-like activity. When it is used in place of regular thromboplastin with factor VII-deficient plasma, a normal clotting time results. The clotting time is prolonged, however, when factor X is deficient. It is available from Burroughs Wellcome Co. and is usually used in a dilution of 1/10,000 (0.5 mg/ml distilled water).

Serum Reagent

Aged serum may be prepared by placing freshly drawn blood into a tube with 2 or 3 glass beads and allowing it to clot. The tube should then be incubated for 4 hours at 37°C. Serum may then be removed after centrifugation and can be further incubated for 24 hours. It can be divided into aliquots and stored in the freezer. To oxalate this serum, add 1 volume sodium oxalate (0.1 M) to 4 volumes serum. Serum reagent is available from Dade, George King, and General Diagnostics. It is used in the differential activated partial thromboplastin time and the differential prothrombin time and can be used in the thromboplastin generation test as a source of normal serum.

Simplastin A

This is a lyophilized preparation of thromboplastin and calcium that contains additional optimal amounts of factors I and V, available from General Diagnostics. It should not be used for the routine screening prothrombin time because deficiencies of factors I and V will not be detected. It may be used in the prothrombin time test on patients receiving oral anticoagulants when the plasma is more than 4 hours old, in the evaluation of a prolonged prothrombin time test, and in the prothrombin consumption test. When the prothrombin time is prolonged with Simplastin A, the defect is most likely a deficiency of factor II, factor VII, factor X, or a combination of these. A circulating anticoagulant could also give an abnormal result with this reagent.

Staphylococcal Clumping Factor

This is available from Sigma Chemical Co. in vials containing 10 mg staphylococcal dried cells. These are stored below 0°C, and after reconstitution with 1 ml distilled water, the suspension is used in the staphylococcal clumping test for fibrinogen-fibrin degradation products. This suspension can be frozen and used again, providing the positive control remains positive.

Thrombin

1. Human thrombin is available commercially as Fibrindex (Ortho). When reconstituted as directed with normal saline, it yields a solution containing 50 U/ml. It can be used in all tests requiring a thrombin solution.
2. Bovine thrombin, topical, is available commercially from Parke-Davis & Co. in vials containing 1000, 5000, and 10,000 units in the lyophilized form. It is convenient to add 10 ml 50% glycerol in barbital-buffered saline to a vial containing 1000 units and then to store this solution in the freezer until ready for use. This gives a stock solution of 100 U/ml. The material can then be withdrawn with a syringe as needed and further diluted to the desired strength with barbital-buffered saline. Thrombin in the 1000-unit vials has proved to be more potent than that in the 5000-unit vials when used in the thrombin time test, and therefore it has been recommended for all tests in this book that require a thrombin solution. Since the quantity is smaller, the material is used up more readily, thus avoiding prolonged storage. The antithrombin III test requires a lower dilution of the 1000-unit thrombin with 5 ml of 50% glycerol in barbital-buffered saline (200 U/ml).

Thromboplastin

Thromboplastin is the term used originally for the coagulant activity of tissue extracts. Many satisfactory tissue extracts of animal brain or lung are available commercially for use primarily in the prothrombin time test. Some are preserved in the liquid state and require mixing with calcium chloride in aliquots. Others are lyophilized and include calcium chloride, being reconstituted with distilled water just prior to use. There are certain differences in these materials, and one particular product should be decided upon and used consistently. It is important to test both normal and abnormal control plasmas daily with the reagent selected.

Urea, 5 Molar

This solution is prepared by dissolving 30 g urea in 100 ml distilled water. The solution is used to test the stability of the clot in the qualitative test for factor XIII.

III. Diagnostic Kits

A variety of kits are available for hemostatic tests. Many of these are described, when applicable, with specific procedures in this book.

IV. Manufacturers of Commonly Used Reagents, Kits, and Instruments

Abbott Laboratories Diagnostics, Chicago, IL

1. A-gent Quantichrome—AT III Kit
2. Platelet Factor$_4$ Radioimmunoassay Diagnostic Kit
3. Quantum I

Aldrich Chemical Co., Inc., Milwaukee, WS

1. Polybrene

Amersham Corp., Arlington Heights, IL

1. β-Thromboglobulin (B-TG) RIA Kit

Becton Dickinson Co. and BBL Microbiology Systems, Cockeysville, MD

1. VACUTAINER tubes, including siliconized tubes
2. Fibrometer
3. ML/ML adapters
4. Needles

Burroughs Wellcome Co., Greenville, NC

1. Thrombo-Wellcotest
2. FDP Kit
3. Russell's viper venom (Stypven)

Bio/Data Corp., Hatboro, PA

1. Coagulation Profiler
2. Platelet Aggregation Profiler
3. Arachidonic acid, collagen, epinephrine, ADP, Aggrecetin, BETA/Pak, PAR/Pak, PAR/Pak II
4. Lyophilized Platelets
5. Fibrinogen Assay Thrombokinetic
6. vW Factor Assay (also, vW abnormal control plasma and vW normal reference plasma

Calbiochem-Behring Corp., LaJolla, CA

1. Antithrombin III Kit (M-Partigen RID plates)
2. Factor VIII-associated protein
3. Plasminogen Kit (M-Partigen RID plates)

Dade Division American Hospital Supply Corp., Miami, FL

1. Protopath (proteolytic enzyme detection system)
   a. Antithrombin III synthetic substrate assay
   b. Heparin synthetic substrate assay
   c. Plasminogen synthetic substrate assay

    d. α_2-antiplasmin synthetic substrate assay
    e.   Prototrol/proteolytic enzyme control
2.   Thromboplastin and activated thromboplastin (prothrombin time (PT) reagents)
3.   Actin—activated cephaloplastin reagent (activated partial thromboplastin time (APTT) reagent)
4.   Adsorbed plasma and serum reagents
5.   Coagulation-factor-deficient substrates
6.   Data-Fi system
    a.   Fibrin(ogen) degradation products (FDP) detection set
    b.   Fibrinogen determination reagents
    c.   Fibrinolysis control
7.   Cluster—platelet aggregation reagents

Diagnostica, Inc., Miami, FL

1.   Glass bead columns
    a.   Adeplat S
    b.   Adeplat T

Eli Lilly and Co., Indianapolis, IN

1.   Protamine sulfate

Gelman Sciences, Inc., Ann Arbor, MI

1.   Electrophoresis equipment and reagents

General Diagnostics, Morris Plains, NJ

1.   Coag-A-Mate instruments
2.   Simplate and Simplate II bleeding-time devices
3.   Simplastin and Simplastin A
4.   Automated APTT reagent
5.   Platelin and Platelin plus Activator (PTT and APTT reagents)
6.   Coagulation-factor-deficient substrates
7.   Correction reagents set
8.   Collagen
9.   Fibrinogen

George King-Bio-Medical Inc., Overland Park, KS

1.   Coagulation-factor-deficient substrates
2.   Assayed normal plasma
3.   Aged serum reagent
4.   Adsorbed plasma reagent
5.   Multi-trait set (Fletcher, Fitzgerald, Passavoy, and von Willebrand)

Helena Laboratories, Beaumont, TX

1.   Ristocetin
2.   Coagulation-factor-deficient substrates
3.   Normal reference plasma (assayed values for all factors)

Kabi Group, Inc., Greenwich, CT

1. Coatest—antithrombin III kit
2. Synthetic chromogenic substrates (for measurement of activity of thrombin, factor X_a, kallikrein, plasmin, and related substances)

Ortho Diagnostic Systems, Inc., Raritan, NJ

1. Thrombofax (PTT reagent)
2. Activated Thrombofax (optimized APTT reagent)
3. Fibrindex (human thrombin)
4. Brain thromboplastin (PT reagent)
5. Antithrombin III assay

Parke-Davis, Detroit, MI

1. Adrenalin Chloride

Pharmacia Fine Chemicals, Inc., Piscataway, NJ

1. Dextran T-10

Potters Industries, Inc., Hasbrouck Heights, NJ

1. Glass beads for platelet retention

Sigma Chemical Co., St. Louis, MO

1. ADP
2. Collagen
3. Staphylococcal clumping factor and diagnostic kit
4. EACA solution
5. Tris-buffered saline
6. Bovine fibrinogen

Index

Page numbers in *italics* refer to illustrations; page numbers followed by t refer to tables.

221